For

all those, like my Karen, who are ill through no fault of their own

there is often a flickering light available on the path to help you

if you are able to see it, please try to use it

DISCLAIMER

This book is not intended to replace the advice of a medical practitioner or to be a substitute.

This is not medical advice and the book is not meant to be used to diagnose bronchiectasis or any other medical condition(s).

The book shares the Author's personal experiences and information about bronchiectasis.

The author has no interest, financial or otherwise, in any equipment or product mentioned in the book and any use of them is the responsibility of the user.

You should take full responsibility for your own health but take cognisance of the input of others.

First published by A. J. Frederick, 2020.

COPYRIGHT

Copyright © Author, A. J. Frederick, 2020.

A.J. Frederick asserts the moral right to be identified as the Author of this work.

All rights reserved. No part of this publication may be reproduced, stored in a retrieval system or elsewhere, or transmitted in any form or by any means; electronic, mechanical, photocopying, recording, scanning or otherwise without written permission of the Author.

It is illegal to copy this book, post it to a website, or distribute it by any other means without permission.

CONTENTS

Acknowledgements

Preface

Introduction to my bronchiectasis journey

CHAPTER 1: SETTING THE SCENE	1
CHAPTER 2: BEING POSITIVE	96
CHAPTER 3: USING ASAFOETIDA ESSENTIAL OIL	117
CHAPTER 4: USING THE PULMONARIA (LUNGWORT) PLANT	159
CHAPTER 5: IMPROVING BREATHING	192
CHAPTER 6: GOOD LIFESTYLE CAN HELP BRONCHIECTASIS	230
CHAPTER 7: POST NASAL DRIP AND BRONCHIECTASIS	262
CONCLUSION	274
APPENDIX: BRONCHIECTASIS RESEARCH	277

ACKNOWLEDGEMENTS

In writing any book, this one included, the Author(s) are usually indebted to a number of people who have helped them either with their researches or in giving their advice on about what has been written. As the sole author of this book I am not an exception to this unwritten rule.

I would therefore like to give thanks to the following people who have helped me;

- My wife Karen who has put up with the (sometimes strangled) vocal sounds I have made in connection with my battles with my computer and its seemingly unfathomable and illogical foibles while I have been writing and producing this book. Also, and more importantly, as the closely involved person who has unfortunately witnessed (and heard) at close proximity, the horrible physical effects of my bronchiectasis

- A great friend of mine, Suzi Rixon who is a highly qualified and experienced healer, Bach Flowers therapist and aromatherapist in Shrewsbury. It was amongst her books that I chanced upon the discovery of the wondrous therapeutic powers of the asafoetida herb. Suzi (and members of her close family) is the epitemy of a rare truly giving person

- Claire Clough of the Rare Books Department of the Library of the Royal Horticultural Society, Vincent Square, London who kindly supplied me with information about asafoetida which is contained in the book 'A new system of agriculture' written by the Rev. John Laurence and published in London in 1726

- Cheryl Kenny, Research networks and partnerships manager at the British Lung Foundation charity who helped with my enquiries about statistics relating to bronchiectasis in the United Kingdom

- Kay Pennick, Wakehurst Place Librarian; Library, Art and Archives, Royal Botanic Gardens Kew, Millennium Seed Bank, Wakehurst, West Sussex who provided information about the accession of seed of Ferula foetida in the MSB at Wakehurst and the propagation of ferula foetida plants gathered from seed, from Kazakhstan and the Kyrgyz republic, at Wakehurst and Kew Gardens, London

- Sue Medway, Director of the Chelsea Physic Garden, Chelsea, London who provided information about ferula asafoetida cultivation, propagation at and seed distribution by the Chelsea Physic Garden

- Brendan Gilsenan, National Botanic Gardens, Glasnevin, Dublin, Eire who informed me about the sources of asafoetida seed which had been supplied to the Botanic Gardens in the past

- Dr Christopher J. Etheridge, Chair BMHA (British Herbal Medicine Association) for patiently answering my queries about pulmonaria and pyrrolizidine alkaloids (PAs) and for setting out the position of his organisation on PAs

- Debra Goodger, Norfolk Essential Oils (www.neoils.com) who supplied information about Asafoetida essential oil

- Ian Carley, Spark Agency, Shropshire ([www.sparkagency.uk)](www.sparkagency.uk) who helped prepare my book for publication and Meryl, also of Spark Agency, for transposing my manuscript into publication format.

PREFACE

Just before I completed this book about bronchiectasis, and my own self-treatment programme for it, the United Kingdom along with most of the rest of the world was struck by the terrible often deadly effects of the Coronavirus (COVID- 19) pandemic. This virus has shone a spotlight on the world of respiratory diseases and conditions and the health disasters experienced by a large number of individuals inflicted with them. These problems can either be short term or lifelong.

I was struck by the fact that bronchiectasis, of all the main respiratory conditions mentioned in the media and by politicians and medical/ scientific experts in relation to COVID -19, has been largely ignored. This is disappointing because worldwide it kills thousands annually in severe cases in 'normal' times. As a pre-existing medical condition, the numbers were probably escalated when COVID struck sufferers.

This bronchiectasis book is about;
- my successful, simple and economical self- help programme and methods which allow me to cope better with my symptoms and have also reduced my reliance on the NHS
- looking at bronchiectasis from a sufferer's perspective
- encouraging people to think about ways that can improve their own respiratory health and lifestyle
- educating people about bronchiectasis, especially how it affects sufferers

- bronchiectasis, the condition – causes, prevention, diagnosis, conventional treatments, numbers affected, research etc.

To help the reader, the book contains;
- ✓ my experiences of having bronchiectasis for over 45 years
- ✓ details about my self-help programme and methods and the usual approaches to this condition (chapters 2 -7)
- ✓ the background to bronchiectasis as it affects both adults and children (chapter 1)
- ✓ questions such as the possible link between bronchiectasis and post nasal drip (chapter 7)
- ✓ a recommendation that people who smoke/vape around babies and toddlers at a time when their lungs are developing should be penalised (chapter 1)
- ✓ details of individual bronchiectasis research and trends (chapter 1) & Appendix
- ✓ the description of bronchiectasis as a 'condition', rather than 'diseased condition' or 'physical disorder'
- ✓ any repetition which occurs, is for emphasis and reinforcement purposes
- ✓ no index, because I have found that in many other non-fiction books there is no completely accurate correlation between an index page listing and what it is purported to relate to – this is both confusing and frustrating for the reader.

Many medical organisations, charities, practitioners and researchers are trying to stimulate debate about bronchiectasis, especially its causes, symptoms and treatment, which for good reason has been described as an 'emerging global epidemic' (source; *Chotirmall & Chalmers,* see chapter 1). Many research papers and reports include a reference to the view that bronchiectasis 'makes a burden on health systems and that this will increase in the future' (sources; chapter 1 & Appendix).

Whilst complementary/ alternative therapies and self-help programmes are often ignored by government and much of the medical profession, the British Thoracic Society stated in the many recommendations contained in its *2019 Guideline for Bronchiectasis in Adults* that;

'further interventional/ randomised controlled trials are needed to establish the role of any alternative therapies in the management of bronchiectasis' (page 6)

'studies assessing the benefits of nutritional supplementation in patients with bronchiectasis should be undertaken' (page 6).

I have read a number of written comments made by leading members in the respiratory field of the medical and therapy professions about the dearth of solid information which exists about bronchiectasis and the treatments used to treat it.

Hopefully;
- ✓ my book, self-help programme and methods will become part of this debate
- ✓ in the future more of the research information about bronchiectasis will become more easily accessible to bronchiectasis sufferers, and other interested

members of the public, at a nominal or no cost (which is often not the current situation).

I hope you enjoy this book, find it interesting and helpful and please remember that lung health can be helped by the sufferer (and his/her supporters) and by members of the medical profession.

Many bronchiectasis sufferers value support, advice and reassurance. I aim to offer these by introducing a personalised subscription internet self-help club based on my Programme and methods. For details, contact bronchiectasisbook@outlook.com. Any information/help given is not intended to replace the advice of a medical practitioner or to be a substitute, or is not to be used to diagnose bronchiectasis or any other medical condition.

A.J.F.

2020

INTRODUCTION TO MY BRONCHIECTASIS JOURNEY

As a long-time bronchiectasis sufferer, I have aimed this book primarily at other sufferers of the condition. They, their family members and probably their friends and colleagues, know only too well that it is a nasty, long term (chronic) respiratory condition with no cure and only management of its symptoms possible. Some preventative actions can ameliorate this condition.

Hopefully, the book's information will also be of interest and help to sufferers of other respiratory conditions.

Having had breathing problems for almost sixty years since childhood, my ongoing chest condition was only diagnosed as bronchiectasis in my local general hospital in Shrewsbury about twenty years ago when a young doctor recognised its signs from a chest CT (Computerised Tomography) scan which looked at my lungs in detail.

After having my long-term respiratory condition finally diagnosed, I thought that there would be a treatment which would either cure or improve it which would be available to me. I had learned to live with a constant cough which made my chest sore and which produced a great deal of phlegm which could vary in colour and consistency from clear through to green (when infection was present); hopefully I thought that these symptoms would become a thing of the past.

I was so disappointed that all that was offered to me, on different occasions, was the prescription of different antibiotics with different strengths to treat my respiratory bacterial infections at different times (Amoxicillin or Doxycycline) depending on the severity of my condition and Carbocisteine which is a mucolytic which allows the sufferer like me to bring up my sputum more easily.

I was worried that the damaging bacteria or pathogen would become increasingly resistant to the antibiotics and that they would also lead to them having harmful side effects.

I was also introduced, during a brief visit to a hospital respiratory physiotherapy department, to a regime which included specific breathing exercises (Active Cycle of Breathing Technique/ ACBT) and a postural drainage method which was designed to clear the lungs of infection through the bringing up of phlegm/ sputum. I had indeed been doing the postural drainage for a long time before the hospital visit.

Having been a complementary therapist for over 30 years I decided to take matters into my own hands and try to develop my own different, self- help treatment programme using methods which would hopefully yield better results to me than what was being offered by the NHS (National Health Service). Before embarking on my own programme, I thought a lot about what could have caused my respiratory problems and my bronchiectasis in particular.

I was brought up in London in the 1950s and 1960s in an age where polluting smogs (a mixture of smoke and fog) were common, sometimes with a reduced field of vision of only a few yards. The polluted air smelt like pure cigarette smoke. Coal fires during this period, using smoky fuel (before the introduction of urban smoke-free zones), were then the norm rather than the clean gas or oil-fired central heating which has been installed in most modern homes and offices.

My mother was a heavy smoker so I was an unwitting passive smoker; at parties, cigarettes in open boxes were freely available to guests! At that time, smoking was fashionable and even de riguer, with most film and sports stars and pop singers being heavy smokers. While my father was not a smoker, he was a life- long tobacco snuff user. This practice had been recommended to him by a doctor in the 1930s to help him clear his nasal passages as they became blocked while doing high board diving at the famous Highgate Lido in North London.

In my teens, I attended a secondary schools' medical clinic (alas, now long gone) in North West London to try to correct my breathing. I always tended to breathe both in and out through my open mouth rather than breathing in through my nose and out through my mouth. I was given exercises to do and I vaguely remember the term 'post nasal drip' being said by one of the clinic's doctors to me.

It was not until I was in my early 20s that I started to develop worse problems with my breathing and my chest. I developed a chronic cough which produced a great deal of mucus/ phlegm which often became infected. I underwent a number of conventional tests to get to the cause of the problem. These ranged from a rudimentary patch test to see if I had any common allergies, to a very unpleasant sinus wash hospital procedure which comprised the cartilage in my nose being broken with the sinus passages then being washed through and then drained (this procedure was both painful and unsuccessful).

As none of my tests proved successful, I had to put up with my undiagnosed condition with only courses of antibiotics and mucolytics being the only treatment offered to me by the NHS. The only practical self-help method I knew about was a physiotherapy style of postural drainage which was designed to drain my lungs of infected phlegm while lying on the side of a bed. This drainage method was helpful only to an extent.

I also tried reducing and then eliminating dairy products as I had read that these helped stimulate the production of mucous. After a month, a non-dairy diet didn't seem to help so I returned to the joys of cheese although for a long while I stayed on soya milk and a cream substitute (which I still use) both of which I found enjoyable.

After my bronchiectasis was diagnosed in my 50s, I was asked whether there was anything I could think of which could have triggered it taking into account my family's medical history. Other than my father's breathing problems during his diving career and my mother's heavy smoking (ironically, at that time she had an office job working for the Chest & Heart Association charity at BMA House in Central London) all I could pinpoint was the possibility of a bacterial infection I might have contracted from sleeping on a camp bed I had used for a couple of nights, in my early 20s, which had come out of storage from a possibly unhealthy damp warehouse.

After my respiratory/breathing problem had been definitely diagnosed as bronchiectasis, for the next ten years I put up with my chronic, productive cough and continued to take different antibiotics when regular infections took hold. My situation was such that I found it embarrassing for both me and my wife who was also long suffering because she had to endure listening to my bouts of prolonged and loud coughing and lung clearing. In addition, my chest was made sore, my throat became sore, I was tired and my antibiotics medication had a bad effect on my digestive processes which became sluggish with painful constipation occurring.

Because my conventional medication didn't seem to be getting to the cause of my condition and only helped temporarily by controlling my symptoms when I had a chest infection, I decided to develop and implement my own self-help methods and a programme to try to better combat and minimise the problems caused by my condition as I had learnt that it was incurable.

In each of the chapters 2 to 7 of this book I have described a specific part of the overall programme and have also given some wider background

information and how it relates to the condition.
Chapter 1 contains bronchiectasis information.

While I have to agree that bronchiectasis cannot be cured in the generally accepted medical sense and its symptoms can only be managed, I have seen concrete positive results in my own experience of this condition since I have been using my methods. These have included;
- ✓ no need to use antibiotics for my condition for the last 5 years (except as an experiment)
- ✓ a marked decrease in the amount of my coughing
- ✓ a reduction of infected phlegm/ sputum
- ✓ a reduction in my use of tissues because of my clearer lungs and nasal area
- ✓ a measured improvement in my breathing which has allowed me to cope better with stressful situations such as when I have to have mouthfuls of water during a lengthy dental treatment
- ✓ an improvement in my sleeping.

My self-help approach has needed hard work and discipline but the financial cost of most component parts of the system I have developed is very low. It could be a possible option to be considered by others but if you want to see if it can supplement your existing medical and therapy treatment it is very advisable that your GP doctor or specialist be consulted and any reduction in medication or change in therapy be done with care and their guidance.

MY SELF-HELP PROGRAMME & METHODS

By deciding to try to help myself instead of using conventional medical aid I introduced a positive philosophical approach into my attempt to get better, especially the reduction of the reliance I may have had on prescribed medication. Part of my positive approach was the desire to reduce my reliance on the use of antibiotics which is the accepted primary medical treatment of bronchiectasis. Unfortunately, as bacteria and pathogens are become increasingly resistant to this type of drug if by minimising my dependence on their use, I hope that if I do have to revert to using them, they will remain effective for me for a longer time.

Possibly the most unusual part of my programme was discovered by chance. It was only when I looked at a friend's aromatherapy book which listed and described the benefits of a herb called asafoetida that I realised that it could possibly provide relief for my own respiratory problem. This herb has been known for thousands of years and is used now throughout the world including the UK mainly for culinary use rather for medicinal purposes.

Countries in the Middle East especially Iran; parts of the Indian subcontinent; Afghanistan and Turkey are the main producers of asafoetida. Traditionally, however, it has been used for medical and agricultural reasons as well as for culinary uses. Asafoetida is valued in Ayurvedic medicine and philosophy.

I decided to use asafoetida in the form of an inhalation of vapours of its essential oil when they are given off after being mixed with hot water. This option was chosen in preference to culinary intake because the vapours are able to enter the respiratory system directly and quickly.

I also wanted to try to see if there was any other natural product I could use which historically had been used to treat respiratory and chest problems. I found a solution in my use of pulmonaria which is a low growing perennial plant commonly found in gardens but also wild in some woods and forests. It has pretty delicate flowers in the spring and distinctively spotted and veined patterned leaves then and thereafter. These spots and veins resemble a view of a lung hence its common English name 'lungwort'.

As it has been used for hundreds, if not thousands, of years to help people with lung problems I thought why not see if it could help me. Instead of eating it raw I decided to use its infused leaves as a form of pleasant tea; after being drunk the leaves can be added to many different dishes and safely eaten.

As I wanted to improve my breathing to see if this would reduce the need for coughing, I devised and regularly used (daily if possible) my own simple breathing improvement system, which I have called the 'Ratio system' which I devised after studying many different breathing methods. Accepting my need to improve my breathing I became a regular user of the sauna at the Castle Country Club, Rowton near

Shrewsbury, Shropshire, with the introduction of Olbas Oil vapour, into its atmosphere, which I inhaled.

As part of my overall full body health & fitness regime I decided to try and improve the action of my lungs and strengthen my chest muscles by concentrating on certain exercises in the gymnasium at Rowton. I also incorporated swimming there into my fitness regime. I did other regular exercises at home in my own gymnasium and used a small, hand held iSmart electronic massager with its 'cupping' action to help relax my back and chest muscles and help loosen mucus.

During the period of lockdown and 'social distancing' during the UK coronavirus (COVID-19) pandemic the health club was shut but as I have made a small home gymnasium, I was able to continue exercising, although I missed the sauna facilities at Rowton. Walking my dogs daily in a local woodland also helped my breathing and my mental health.

As I have previously mentioned in this foreword, it was thought that I suffered from a medical condition called Post Nasal Drip. When I examined the consistency and colour of the seemingly non-infected mucus which sometimes was expelled from my lungs it seemed to resemble that which was produced from my nasal and sinus areas. I thought that gravity must lead to some of the fluid originating from these two relatively small facial/ skull spaces entering the lungs. Logically, I thought therefore that if I could devise a method to reduce the volume of liquid which was dripping, this should reduce my coughing and the amount of mucus which is produced in my airways and lungs. I also devised a couple of simple physical methods of clearing my nasal and sinus cavities.

By reducing my coughing and mucus I thought this could have the added benefit of reducing the stress on my body and mind brought about by my condition.

CONCLUSION

I have given the reader the background to the reasons, why and how, I devised my own self-help programme and methods to help me greatly reduce the problems caused by the symptoms of my medically diagnosed bronchiectasis. This reduction has been successful for me but as bronchiectasis is a respiratory problem which affects people individually, it is important that everyone looks at their own situation.

If anyone does decide to try my programme and methods, they will need discipline and determination to follow it properly and hopefully win through wholly or partly with an improvement in the bronchiectasis. At least there are no expensive clinics or courses to attend, exorbitantly expensive supplements to take or complicated diets to follow.

I realise that there are differing degrees of this horrible condition but as It worked for me you could consider whether it could help you.

However, please STOP if you experience any worsening of your condition's symptoms which can be directly attributed to trying any of my methods.

Best wishes and good luck on your health improvement journey.

A. J. Frederick
2020

CHAPTER 1: SETTING THE SCENE

The Aims of this chapter are;

1. to give the reader information about bronchiectasis
2. to give a brief description of respiration, and the organs and structures which affect it.

Bronchiectasis is a progressive chronic (long term) non-contagious, inflammatory diseased lung condition (the 'condition'), which often worsens over time. This pathological process wreaks immune- infective- inflammatory irreversible lung and lower airways destruction which leads to a terrible cycle of (often frequently) repeated periods when lung health gets worse (exacerbations). It is one of the different chronic suppurative lung diseases (CSLD) which 'fester' and form 'pus'.

Although it is generally considered to be non-reversible, the progression of mild bronchiectasis as determined by radiography might be slowed or halted at any age if it is treated early and the lung function decline associated with its progression can also be halted. The management of its symptoms is one of the key ways of treating it. Details about reports on the reversibility of the effects of bronchiectasis and the importance of early diagnosis are given later (page 67) in this chapter.

Bronchiectasis can directly and adversely affect the quality of life of adults, children and the young who suffer from it and indirectly their family members and others. It is a significant condition because it can cause premature death (source: *Deinfort DP et al 'Bronchiectasis in Central Australia: a young face to an old disease' Respir Med 2008; 102: 1521-1528*). Bronchiectasis mortality rates vary greatly between different countries.

In this chapter we look at current thinking about bronchiectasis in both adults and children/young people and we consider;

- what is bronchiectasis?
- international research
- causes
- symptoms
- diagnosis
- conventional medical treatment and sufferers' self-help techniques.

The human respiratory/breathing process is a wondrous thing and the lungs and their action are only part of this process.

Other organs and parts of the body which are part of, and affect, this process are;

- the brain
- the nose, mouth and the facial sinuses
- the airway between the nose and the trachea
- the trachea
- the lungs
- the diaphragm muscle and the chest muscles.

WHAT IS BRONCHIECTASIS?

The word bronchiectasis is derived from the Greek word 'Bronkos' meaning bronchial/ airway and 'ectasis' meaning widening.

Bronchiectasis has a radiological or pathological diagnosis characterised by an abnormal and permanent bronchi dilation; this diagnosis is made mostly by a chest high-resolution computed tomography (c-HRCT) scan which is the current diagnostic gold standard. In addition, there is the clinical syndrome of cough, sputum production and/ or recurrent respiratory infections to be taken into account in relation to diagnosis.

It is more accurately described as a pathologic condition rather than disease and while it is often pre – fixed with the description 'non-cystic fibrosis (CF), there is no identifiable pathological difference to that found in cystic fibrosis.

It arises from an infection and an ineffective host immune response involving uncontrolled recruitment and activation of inflammatory cells within the lower airways in the lungs. There is a subsequent release of mediator cells, such as proteases (enzymes) and free radicals (atoms/ groups of atoms which damage cells) which cause injury to the bronchial walls and their consequent dilation (widening).

One or both bronchi (the air passages leading into the lungs from the trachea) become abnormally distorted and stretched (ectasis) wider than normal and have their linings damaged. This physical situation will then leave the way open for the condition's pathological process to proceed. It destroys the muscular and elastic components of the walls of the airways and is worst if it occurs in early childhood before the respiratory tract is fully developed.

It can occur in part of a lung or in the whole lung and It affects one or both lungs. It is in the damaged part of the lung(s) that more mucus is produced than in the unaffected part of the lung.

The management and minimisation of its symptoms and taking actions which can prevent its symptoms have been the main traditional medical approach. Self- management, especially if it incorporates a planned approach with goals and outcomes, should comprise an active partnership between the sufferer/patient and involved health professionals.

Bronchiectasis can affect sufferers both physically and psychologically. Physically, its symptoms such as continual coughing, expelling mucus by spitting out and tiredness can lead to psychological effects such as frustration and embarrassment when in the company of others.

Bronchiectasis is one of the most neglected respiratory diseases and it has no clear classifications. Little is known about its prevalence (number of cases) especially in Asia where it appears in an aggressive form. Asian prevalence is higher than that in Europe and North America. Because it appears that the incidence (number of new cases annually) is increasing it has been described by researchers Chotirmall S. H. & Chalmers J.D *(source: Article in BMC Pul Med 18, 76 (22 May 2018))* as an emerging 'global epidemic'.

Bronchiectasis affects all age groups from children through to those of retirement years. Congenital (present from birth) bronchiectasis only affects children whereas non-congenital bronchiectasis typically affects adults and older children. Its symptoms range from mild to severe and its severity can now be scored using either of two different systems (the Bronchiectasis Severity Index and the FACED Score), these systems are described later in this chapter).

Within the two lungs, the bronchi divide again and again into thousands of smaller airways called bronchioles. With bronchiectasis, these too can become scarred and inflamed with thick mucus which cannot clear themselves properly. Mucus will then build up and the airways can get infected by bacteria and other pathogens. Small pockets in the airways mean that the trapped mucus is likely to get infected; this pattern of infection can recur.

Bronchiectasis is characterised by chronic coughing, sputum production and 'vicious cycles' (a description based on *P.J. Cole's 1962 'Vicious Cycle Hypothesis'*) of often debilitating recurring infections (also known as flare-ups or exacerbations). These can lead to a damaging progressive loss of lung function which leads to chronic morbidity(disease) and in severe instances, premature death. It is also characterised by a cycle of drug (normally antibiotics) and physiotherapy treatment regimes.

A bronchiectasis flare-up or exacerbation has been defined in the British Thoracic Society (BTS) guidelines as 'an acute deterioration in the nature of the cough with increased sputum volume, purulence (*discharge of pus*) and viscosity (*thickness or stickiness*)'. (Italics are the author's additions).

CAUSES OF BRONCHIECTASIS

There are a number of causes of bronchiectasis and the most common is a previously acute lung infection which can have happened during childhood or as a young adult. This, and the many other causes of bronchiectasis, which can coexist (comorbidity) with other medical conditions are covered later in this chapter.

Whilst there are a number of causes of bronchiectasis, up to 50% of cases (children and adults) have no known (idiopathic) cause.

Bronchiectasis is often a complication of cystic fibrosis (CF) which is an inherited disease, one of the results of which is that the glands in the lining of the airways produce thick mucus. If it is not diagnosed and treated early then any condition such as pneumonia, bronchiectasis or bronchitis can develop and lung damage occur.

When bronchiectasis develops, with its damage to one or both airways (bronchi), the process of one of the body's natural defences is disturbed. This defence process is the normal production of a small amount of mucus (also called phlegm or sputum), by tiny glands in the lining of the airways, that keeps the airways moist and traps any dust, dirt and germs which are breathed in. This process is repeated within the lungs which contain the smaller airways called bronchioles, which lead away, and divide, from the bronchi. Phlegm is the specific name for mucus which is coughed up from the lungs. The colour of phlegm varies depending on the lungs' condition and it different for each person at different times.

There is a difference in composition between mucus and sputum. Mucus is a viscoelastic gel comprised of water, mucins (which are glycoproteins) serum, cellular proteins and lipids/fatty acids. Sputum is expectorated mucus together with inflammatory cells, cellular debris, DNA and bacteria.

As we have seen, bronchiectasis causes structural lung changes including an abnormal widening of the bronchi and bronchioles airways. These airways become scarred and inflamed with extra thickened mucus building up and pooling in parts of the widened airways which cannot clear themselves properly. The airways will then become infected by bacteria and this build- up of plugged, retained bacteria will inflame and further damage the airways. Pockets in the airways will develop in which mucus is trapped and infection is intensified and there is the possibility of emphysema developing.

Bacteria can stick to mucus and this proliferation gives a large bacteria count in the sputum. Bronchiectasis sputum can be more purulent and adhesive compared with other chronic respiratory diseases such as COPD (Chronic Obstructive Respiratory Disease).

Bronchiectasis inflammation is primarily linked to neutrophil white cell activity and persistent bacterial infection. This inflammation is due to increased exacerbation frequency. Rapid lung function decline is because of degradation of airway elastin and other mechanisms. There are also other cells such as T-cells which play their part.

The normal process of clearing mucus secretions is primarily by the normal action of the MCC (Mucociliary Clearance/ Mucociliary escalator) body defence system, which covers most of the nose, bronchi and bronchioles, especially by the action of ciliary hair movement.

This action can be impaired by the impact of the structural bronchiectasis and a combination of one or more of the following conditions - airway dehydration; absence of lubricant activity which prevents adhesion of mucus to airways surfaces; inherent defects within the cilia, specific antibody deficiencies and the viscosity and volume of excess mucus which is being produced.

With healthy people the cilia propel mucus up the airway at a rate of 4/5 mm per minute. With MCC there is a co-ordinated and synchronised beating of the cilia across multiple ciliated cells. This process is disrupted, as in the case of bronchiectasis, if the mucus load it carries becomes excessive.

It is thought that the lack of motile (moveable) cilia associated with bronchiectasis could be due to the lack of a key protein (IFT protein 88, encoded by the IFT88 gene) as depletion of this protein decreases cilia beat frequency.

Usually between 20-30ml of secretions are produced in the airway by the MCC daily and swallowed. If the amount of mucus exceeds this amount, a cough is needed to clear the mucus in the airway.

The rate of clearance is influenced by mucus hydration and its state, rigidity and viscosity. This situation points to the need to drink the necessary amount of fluid, especially water.

The secondary process in clearing mucus (and inhaled irritants) is the cough mechanism which is initiated by inflammatory, chemical, mechanical or thermal stimulation of receptors which are found within the respiratory system from the oropharynx down to the lung. The involuntary or voluntary cough is in three parts; firstly, an inspiratory gasp; secondly, glottis closing which traps air in the lungs and narrows the trachea and bronchi; finally, sudden glottis opening causing air to explode violently upwards so shearing secretions off the airway walls.

With bronchiectasis causing structural changes and damage to the lung(s) including bronchial dilation, wall thickening and mucus plugging the result can be small airways disease, the reduction of the cough mechanism's efficiency and possibly emphysema. This further wall damage, continued infections and perpetual inflammatory responses become a vicious circle'.

An excellent illustrated explanation and description of the body's defence system in the airways and alveolus in contained in the Australian *Bronchiectasis Toolbox* website:
http://www.bronchiectasis.com.au/physiotherapy/principles-of-airway-clearance/airway-clearance-in-the-normal-lung

The aetiology (cause or causes) of bronchiectasis can help understand the primary causes of the disease i.e. is it post infective or immune deficiency.

In the past, childhood chest infections which could have led to bronchiectasis, such as measles, whooping cough, tuberculosis (TB) or bacterial infections were more prevalent. As these conditions have largely been controlled by immunisation and antibiotic drugs their incidence has fallen dramatically. The importance of having vital childhood and adult immunisations cannot be stressed enough.

If children are affected by the results of early chronic infections these may persist later into adulthood. As with adults, there are different degrees of severity of this condition. Older people, as well as children, can also develop severe lung conditions which affect or damage airways that can cause bronchiectasis.

Chronic airways Infection, most frequently with *Haemophilus influenzae* bacterium and *Pseudomonas aeruginosa* and less frequently with other organisms stimulate and sustain lung inflammation with an increased exacerbation frequency, worse quality of life and increased mortality. This is especially significant with *P. aeruginosa* which has been associated with a 3- fold mortality risk, almost 7- fold increase in risk of hospital admission and an average additional exacerbation per patient annually (*Source: Ann Am Thorac Soc 2015; 12: 1602-1611*).

It has been estimated that 30% of bronchiectasis sufferers are infected with the *H. influenzae* bacterium. In Israel, research has shown that those aged 64 and younger are more likely to be infected with *H. influenzae* and those over 64 are more likely to be infected with *P. aeruginosa* and *Enterobacteriaceae*.

Other conditions, that affect or damage airways, which can cause bronchiectasis include;

- some inherited conditions such as primary ciliary dyskinesia which affect the normal structure or function of the lungs or the airways' hair-like cilia so that they don't move correctly to clear the airways; or cystic fibrosis
- chronic obstructive pulmonary disease (COPD) or asthma

- bacteria, such as the bacterium *Pseudomonas aeruginosa* (about 16% of cases)
- post - infection, including tuberculosis (TB) and non-tuberculosis mycobacterial (NTM), whooping cough or pneumonia, can damage the airways at time of infection
- NTM together with the presence of *P. aeruginosa* correlate with severe disease, worse lung function and more frequent exacerbations. This lung disease is common in the USA and parts of Asia
- studies of species of fungi such as *Aspergillus fumigatus,* which develop in the mucus-rich lungs, are indicating that they may be pathogens responsible for the condition. *A. fumigatus* fungus and its spores are found in the soil, plants, household dust & in the air
- inflammatory bowel disease which is also called ulcerative colitis and Crohn's disease
- immune system deficiencies, which mean that bacterial infections are more likely to happen (especially in children). An example of an immune deficiency, is the presence of the *Pregnancy zone protein (PZP)* which powerfully suppresses the immune system
- arthritis disorders
- airways becoming blocked by an inhaled object such as a nut which becomes stuck; this may lead to local damage to that airway. Abscesses can also lead to obstructions
- regurgitated acid ('reflux') from the stomach that is inhaled, can damage airways as well as leading to the inhalation of poisonous gases. This is more

common in children because their food tube/ oesophagus is shorter.

SYMPTOMS OF BRONCHIECTASIS

Bronchiectasis symptoms are caused by;

- chronic bronchial infections
- inflammation
- impaired mucociliary clearance of inhaled particles and pathogens before they reach the lungs
- existing structural lung damage.

Symptoms vary from person to person and also at different times. Sometimes they will be mild, sometimes moderate and at other times they will be severe.

When mild, occasional coughing up small amounts of clear or light-coloured sputum happens and there are infrequent chest infections. When severe, large amounts of dark yellow/ green/ brown sputum are coughed up on most days. When moderate, symptoms are between mild and severe.

Phlegm (or sputum) is produced only in the mucus membranes which line the respiratory system. It is not produced in the nasal or sinus cavities but in the tracheal tube and within the lungs. In contrast, mucus is produced from the mucus glands of the mucus membranes which are found in many systems of the body. Phlegm is thicker than mucus and unlike mucus it may have colour. The function of both secretions is protective and their constituents are similar.

The colour of phlegm varies depending on the lungs' condition and it different for each person but generally;

- white or clear phlegm/ sputum produced every now or then is normal
- yellow or green phlegm indicates infection – cold, flu or chest infection. Green phlegm is more likely to be a bacterial infection than a yellow phlegm
- streaked red phlegm indicates blood due to a lot of heavy of severe coughing (haemoptysis) which has damaged blood vessel walls which leak.

With bronchiectasis, chest infection is almost permanent and bacteria are found in the person's sputum even when he/she is feeling well. These infections are associated with inflammation of the airways and the respiratory system. More severe and frequent exacerbations are associated with worse quality of life, daily symptoms, decline in lung function and mortality. About 50% of European bronchiectasis sufferers have two or more exacerbations annually and 33% need hospitalisation (source: *ERJ Open Res 2016; 2: 00081-2015*).

The main result of bronchiectasis chronic lung infection (which is usually recurring) is a cough which is associated with the production of clear or coloured sputum/phlegm.

Other symptoms which can occur are;

❖ having difficulty breathing or feeling short of breath especially when exercising, which is caused by

obstructed airflow, impaired gas transfer, lack of activity and comorbidities
- ❖ feeling tired or having difficulty in concentrating
- ❖ chest or joint pain
- ❖ a crackling mid-inspiratory sound, which is caused by air being forced through narrowed airways which are the result of inflammation, secretions or oedema/ excessive fluid accumulation
- ❖ problems with the facial sinuses and/ or nasal passages
- ❖ anxiety or depression
- ❖ cough incontinence, which is also known as bladder leakage
- ❖ possible bad breath/ halitosis
- ❖ coughing up blood which is usually caused by either a chest infection which gives small amounts of blood or by the erosion of blood vessels in the bronchi which gives larger amounts. Occasionally it is the result of another lung condition
- ❖ thickening of the skin under the toe and/or finger nails ('clubbing') it is a sign of fluid accumulation and whilst cause is not definite, it could be related to protein levels.

The effects of short and long- term infections on bronchiectasis

Short term infections such as pneumonia or flu while not directly causing bronchiectasis can cause weak spots or ulcers in the bronchial walls. It is advisable to have an annual flu jab to vaccinate against pneumococcal infection. It may also be helpful to take a vitamin D supplement and eating food rich in vitamin D (including oily fish, white meat and egg yolk) if its level is low.

Long term infections can cause the continued inflammation of these bronchial walls. The elastic muscle fibres degenerate and this facilitates the dilation of the bronchi. When dilation occurs, this leads to any secretions present to build up; infection spreads and intensifies.

Empirical understanding of bronchiectasis, its antibiotics treatment and recent research

Up until recent times there has been a culture of underestimating the significance of bronchiectasis in its prevalence (number of cases), incidence (number of new cases), mortality and an analysis of those affected. This has been important, because in the past it has been considered as an 'orphan' medical condition with a relatively small number of sufferers.

There have been a number of recent reports, papers and articles about bronchiectasis and its antibiotics treatments produced in different countries such as the UK, the USA, Germany, South Korea, Catalonia (Spain), Australia and New Zealand and the statistics and findings in these reports dispute many existing assumptions about bronchiectasis and its treatment.

More details about some of this research will be found in the Appendix at the end of this book.

By accepting previous thinking on this matter, many governments and their health departments have not implemented appropriate policies and forward planning to cater for the actual greater number, and types, of sufferers than previously thought.

Common themes contained in reports about bronchiectasis

There are a number of common themes in many bronchiectasis reports and these include;

- mortality rates for bronchiectasis sufferers of both sexes were much higher than in the general population
- although bronchiectasis is generally not as well-known as some other respiratory conditions such asthma, cystic fibrosis, and TB, more people in the UK die from the condition and its mortality rate has risen by 36% in the UK between 2008 and 2012 (source: British Lung Foundation, www.statistics.blf.org.uk/lung-disease-uk-big-picture). More information in the Appendix.
- data on the coexistence of bronchiectasis with other diseases is lacking but necessary to help inform health management and allocate healthcare resources
- additional research is needed to identify the reasons for increased prevalence/ number of cases and to promote education about bronchiectasis

- across all age groups and both sexes, bronchiectasis increased except in men and women aged 80 plus
- more women than men had bronchiectasis
- bronchiectasis was more common in patients with higher socioeconomic status
- a majority of people had at least one cooccurring and coexisting comorbid condition; in ranking - asthma, COPD, HIV positive, rheumatoid arthritis, connective tissue disorders and ABPA (allergic bronchopulmonary aspergillosis, which is caused by a common mould)
- bronchiectasis has a wide range of causes and associated comorbidities
- mortality rates in adults with bronchiectasis varied widely nationally; 58% survival at 4 years (Turkey), 75% at 8.8 years (Finland), 81% at 14 years (Scotland) (source: *report by Loebinger M.R. et al, Eur Res Journal 2009 34: 843-849*)
- the clinical importance of bronchiectasis is increasing in all aspects of bronchiectasis – actual incidence and rate of incidence, prevalence, hospital admissions and mortality which is an increasing *'burden'* (author's italics) on public health financial and other costs
- patients with bronchiectasis spent more time in hospital and have a higher annual medical care expenditure than age and sex- matched controls with other chronic illnesses such as diabetes and heart failure (source: Weycker D et al *'Prevalence and economic burden of bronchiectasis pub Clin. Pulm Med 2005; 12: 205-209)*

- there is an increase in the rate of first diagnosis; in the UK for instance this increased from 20 per 100,000 people in 2004 to 33 per 100,000 in 2012 (source; British lung Foundation)
- the prevalence and incidence of bronchiectasis is substantially higher than earlier reports indicated, highlighting the importance of obtaining better epidemiological studies and data, diligent surveillance and attentive treatment of this condition.

DIAGNOSIS OF BRONCHIECTASIS

Early diagnosis of bronchiectasis in adults, children and young people is most important because delays of years, or decades of years, which has happened in the past has led to many people (like the author!) being undiagnosed and untreated even if they have had a wet/ productive cough for several years. This situation has led to more preventable damage being done to the lungs and the respiratory system and its functioning, and the risk of premature and accelerated pulmonary and respiratory decline.

Early diagnosis and appropriate treatment and, if possible, prevention of bronchiectasis will help the sufferer in many different ways. but the condition has had, and will have increasingly in the future, a profound effect on most country's health resources and finances. Patients for example in the USA were found to spend two more days in hospital and have a higher annual medical care expenditure (US$5,681) than age and sex- matched controls with other chronic illnesses such as diabetes and heart failure (source: Weycker D et al *'Prevalence and economic burden of bronchiectasis pub Clin. Pulm Med 2005; 12: 205-209).*

Unfortunately, bronchiectasis can be misdiagnosed as, or coexist along with, other chronic respiratory diseases (comorbidities). Examples of this are the number of people who have COPD or difficult- to- control asthma and a chronic cough as well as bronchiectasis. The effects of complications and these bronchiectasis- associated comorbidities extend beyond the respiratory system and include cardiac and/ or psychological problems. In addition, if bronchiectasis is misdiagnosed as asthma then it is likely that the patient will have responded poorly to asthma therapies, which is not surprising as these are inappropriate.

The diagnosis routes

The GP (Primary Health Doctor)

Bronchiectasis diagnosis is usually made by a doctor's assessment of symptoms such as the nature of the patient's cough (wet or dry); whether there are other respiratory symptoms; and exercise tolerance. A detailed patient history will include the frequency and severity of chest infections; the reaction to medications such as antibiotics, bronchodilators and mucolytics; and hospital admissions due to respiratory causes.

A family medical history will be taken and if family members have similar symptoms this may suggest conditions such as Cystic fibrosis (CF) or Primary Ciliary Dyskinesia (PCD}. It is important to know if there has been exposure to smoke, especially tobacco smoke, at home or work or at leisure.

If it is thought that a patient has bronchiectasis, he/she will be referred to a hospital to be seen there by a consultant (or member of his/ her team).

Hospital tests

A chest X-ray and if necessary, a more sophisticated (c)HRCT ((chest) high resolution computerised tomography) scan are taken in the hospital's radiology department and then evaluated at the hospital to see if the airways are widened.

Although the lung's airways and the sputum contained in them, do not normally show up on a standard chest X-ray this may be the case if their walls are thickened. Generally however, the X-ray will appear to be normal or near- normal in patients suspected of suffering from bronchiectasis and even when the results are abnormal, the changes which are present may not obviously be due to bronchiectasis.

Other lung function, sputum and blood tests help to give a more accurate picture of the condition of the lung(s) especially the extent of the damage to the bronchi and to find out if any, and type of, bacterium or another pathogen is present. All of these tests help to confirm the diagnosis of the condition and whether it is bronchiectasis or not.

Sometimes a bronchoscopy (using a camera in a narrow tube to look inside your lungs and take samples) will be carried out.

Specialised breathing tests

Various breathing and lung function tests can be used to help diagnose bronchiectasis and to assess aspects of breathing. These tests include spirometry, FVC (Forced Vital Capacity), FEV1 (Forced Expiratory Volume in one second) and PEF (Peak Expiratory Flow). The GP or consultant will be able to fully explain the tests and their results, including degrees of severity of the condition, to a patient whose respiratory health is being tested.

Genetic blood tests and upper airways tests

If necessary, further tests such as genetic blood tests will be used to try to determine the cause of bronchiectasis. If it is suspected that the bronchiectasis symptoms are linked to chronic rhinosinusitis or upper airway symptoms, tests will be carried out using a nasal endoscopy or an HRCT scan of the sinuses.

Immunological and bacterial/ pathogen tests

Sufferers should be blood sample tested for a condition called Allergic Bronchopulmonary Aspergillosis (ABPA) which is caused by a common mould.

Specialised immunological tests are required in a small proportion of patients with bronchiectasis to make a diagnosis of primary immune deficiency. Clinicians should be aware that some laboratory tests of immune function are not quality assured and that definite guidelines of diagnosis of primary immune deficiencies may be modified as the understanding of the immune system increases (source: *British Thoracic Society (BTS) Bronchiectasis Guideline – consultation March 2018, page 5*). It would seem from this BTS document which reviews 45 international reports into the causes of, and investigations into, bronchiectasis *that much research work needs to be done in the United Kingdom.*

When sputum samples are analysed, they may indicate the presence of different bacteria or other pathogens and their isolation and sensitivity will recommend the most appropriate antibiotic to use. There are many common organisms including; *pseudomonas aeruginosa, haemophilus influenzae, MAC (Myobacterium avium complex, which consists of two similar bacteria found in soil & dust) and staphylococcus aureus.*

In adults, the *Pseudomonas aeruginosa* and *Haemophilus influenzae* pathogens are the most common; in children they are the *H. influenzae, Strep. Pneumoniae* and *Moraxella catarrhalis.*

Many airway samples fail to show the growth of pathogenic bacteria. As the condition worsens, the flora can change with *P. aeruginosa* appearing which can give a predicted worse prognosis.

Aspergillus and *NTM* species are detected in some adults and NTM has been implicated in exacerbations occurring and pulmonary deterioration.

Signs of advanced bronchiectasis

There are several signs of advanced bronchiectasis and these include;

- more than 3 courses of antibiotics per year
- bacteria regularly in the sputum
- a hospital admission because of bronchiectasis in the last year
- walking limited to 100 metres because of breathlessness
- breathless when washing and dressing.

Recognising and assessing flare-ups/ exacerbations

A bronchiectasis flare-up or exacerbation happens when symptoms get worse over a few days and this is usually due to a chest infection. The GP should be contacted as quickly as possible if there are any changes in any of the following;

- feeling unwell
- increased breathlessness
- increased coughing
- increased tiredness and listlessness
- change of sputum colour to green
- increase in the amount or thickness of sputum being produced
- blood in the sputum.

When a sufferer is having a bronchiectasis flare-up, measurements can be taken to assess its extent. These include using a pulse oximeter for blood haemoglobin (haemoglobin)/ oxygen saturation (SATS) level & pulse rate; a thermometer for body temperature (normal = 37°C/ 98.4°F) and a blood pressure monitor. It is always a good idea to discuss the readings with a GP or consultant as there are many variables e.g. age or sex, to take into account.

Monitoring of bronchiectasis and its treatment

If bronchiectasis sufferers are routinely monitored by a health care professional (normally a GP) this will identify its progression and any pathogen emergence. This will enable an existing treatment plan to be modified if necessary.

The frequency of the routine monitoring will vary depending on the condition's severity but it should be done annually and more frequently in worse cases. A sputum sample will be analysed, bodyweight and BMI recorded and a review of flare - ups made. A flare-up has the symptoms of feeling unwell and the coughing up of more sputum with a possible change in colour and increased breathlessness which occur for more than 48 hours.

A plan should be agreed with the health professional about what to do when symptoms start to flare-up. Precautionary stand- by antibiotics which are kept at home can be used.

Bronchiectasis levels scoring systems

The Bronchiectasis Severity Index (BSI)

The BSI is a predictive tool developed in the UK, Belgium and Italy which helps to estimate mortality and hospitalisation rates of bronchiectasis patients. It is also predictive of exacerbations and quality of life giving a broad assessment of the severity of the condition. It could also be a guide to helping decisions about the frequency and intensity of follow-ups and the use of chronic antibiotic treatment.

The scores are calculated incorporating nine variables such as age, BMI, %FEV1 Predicted, previous hospital admissions, number of exacerbations in previous year, MMRC (UK Modified Medical Research Council) breathlessness/ dyspnoea score, *Pseudomonas* colonisation, colonisation with other organisms and radiological severity. The scores are ranked to indicate a mild, moderate or severe level of bronchiectasis.

The calculations' results should not be used on their own to guide clinical care and are not a substitute for clinical judgements. It is a tool that identifies patients at risk of future mortality, hospitalisation and exacerbations.

The FACED score

This Faced score, which was developed in Spain, is a simple predictive bronchiectasis tool which scores the severity of people suffering with non- cystic fibrosis bronchiectasis based on five variables – age, clinical aspects (dyspnoea/ difficult or laboured breathing), lung function (FV1), microbiology (chronic bronchial infection by *Pseudomonas aeruginosa* pathogen) and CT radiological findings (number of affected lobes detected in a computed tomography scan).

It was very successful in accurately predicting all-cause and respiratory mortality, dividing patients into mild, moderate and severe groups according to disease; bronchiectasis mortality and morbidity (the rate of disease) rates; patients with severe exacerbations; and those with more frequent and relevant exacerbations. Again, the score is a tool for assisting clinicians in their assessment and treatment of their patients.

When the results of the BSI and FACED were compared by Mlnov J *et al* in *The Open Respiratory*

Medicine Journal (2015; 9: 46-51) the authors found similar results regarding the assessment of severity by both tools.

Problems about getting tested and treated in UK hospitals

According to the British Thoracic Society website (www.brit-thoracic.org.uk) of 4 December 2019 there are a number of worrying statistics and trends in hospitals related to lung problems which obviously include bronchiectasis. These include;

- number of lung illness attendances at English hospital A & E departments more than doubled between 2010/11 and 2018/19
- lung problems are the main cause of 'excess winter deaths' in A & E departments
- 50% of UK hospitals in 2019 had at least one respiratory consultant post vacancy, up by 10% since 2015
- 50% of respiratory nurses plan to retire or are eligible for retirement within the next 10 years
- lung specialists are under undue pressure which leads to patients experiencing longer waits for hospital out- patient appointments
- lung specialists are experiencing 'burn out'
- a number of hospital lung services are running with a limited physiology workforce which is necessary to delivering and interpreting diagnostic tests such as lung function tests.

With the pressure on thoracic health workers dealing with people suffering during the COVID-19 pandemic in 2020 in hospitals and elsewhere this situation has been greatly exacerbated.

TREATMENTS OF BRONCHIECTASIS

Damage to the lungs and airways caused by bronchiectasis will be permanent and irreversible. However, treatment and management of its symptoms can be done and they should;

- ✓ be able to prevent further progressive lung damage and preserve its function
- ✓ prevent, reduce and suppress acute and chronic bronchial/ chest infections and flare-ups/ exacerbations
- ✓ reduce and control symptoms such as coughing, clearing mucus and tiredness
- ✓ prevent mucus clogging up the airways which are reducing airflow
- ✓ make it easier to live with, so improving the sufferer's quality of life
- ✓ prevent secondary complications such as reduced lung function and the coughing up of blood (haemoptysis)
- ✓ achieve a balance between the potential beneficial effects of intervention against the burden of treatment and the risk of adverse effects from it.

The main medicinal treatment for bronchiectasis is the use of antibiotic drugs which help control infections, but not the continual inflammation which may be progressively destroying the airways. Other types of drug are aimed at reducing the amount of sputum which is produced and to help it be expelled more easily. Specialised respiratory physiotherapy is the main therapeutic treatment for bronchiectasis.

The overall management of bronchiectasis should be seen as two separate but linked, approaches. The first is utilising existing conventional medication and therapy intervention and the other is a sufferer taking responsibility for his/ her own self-help regime which can involve guidance from professionals in the field.

Medical and therapy interventions

Antibiotic drugs and macrolide, mucoactive, mucolytic and mucroregulating medications

Antibiotics

An antibiotic is a type of medicine/ drug that inhibits or destroys microorganisms and fights and prevents bacterial infection.

Because bronchiectasis arises from infection with a subsequent release of certain enzymes and free radicals which cause bronchial-wall injury and damage it is necessary to reduce the microbial load to mitigate the damage. This is achieved by administering intensive, suitable, individualised antibiotic drug treatments.

The most common method of medically treating and controlling a chest infection or a bronchiectasis flare-up (exacerbation), which is caused by an infective organism, is a course, or courses, of antibiotic drugs (often for up to 14 – 21 days). These can vary in strength depending on the individual's needs and the condition's severity at any time. It is important for the patient to finish the course as often they only provide maximum effect at its conclusion.

Evidence about the duration of a course has been questioned and sometimes a course may last only 7 days. The duration may depend on whether things change in the nature of the condition. A sputum sample should be given to a GP or hospital consultant (or member of his/her team) so that guidance can be given at the start of a treatment or when consideration can be given to changing to a different antibiotic.

A patient may be offered long term antibiotics if three or more infections happen yearly. Self- clearance of sputum from the lungs should reduce the number of infections and also any coughing. Often the patient will keep a supply of antibiotics at home in case a flare-up occurs or a GP is not available to be consulted (directly or over the phone).

In the United Kingdom, the standard antibiotics to treat flare-ups or chest infection are either Amoxicillin, or Clarithromycin (for people who are allergic on penicillin); either of which can be usually be taken for a 14-day course. Other tablet antibiotics available are doxycycline, ciproflaxin, coamoxiclav or azithromycin.

While most sufferers are able to take antibiotics, which have been prescribed by the GP (after possible liaison with a respiratory consultant) without staying as an inpatient in hospital they can be treated under ambulatory care (where medical care is provided on an outpatient hospital basis).

If it is necessary to be given antibiotics intravenously (directly into a vein) this may be done in a hospital. In hospital a course will normally last two weeks. If the patient finds it more convenient, and is capable, this can be learnt to be done at home, possibly by a community nurse if a local service can be accessed by the patient. There will always be support offered by the hospital.

If a patient is hospitalised, intravenous antibiotics may be combined with intensive physiotherapy together with other airway clearance methods including nebulised therapy when antibiotics such as gentamicin or colomycin are delivered via a mist through a nebuliser mask.

Positive responses to antibiotic treatment include a reduction in sputum volume and purulence (infection, putridity etc); improvement in cough characteristics such as improving from wet to dry to cessation; reduced inflammation; improved general wellbeing and quality of life; and return to original state of health.

On the negative side, there is a risk of antibiotic resistance; and some nebulised drugs are poorly tolerated.

Macrolide antibiotic drugs

Macrolide is a class of antibiotic drugs which is derived from erythromycin which was originally synthesised from a natural product (a soil bacterium called *Streptomyces erythraeus*). Later drugs were synthesised from erythromycin and they include clarithromycin, azithromycin and roxithromycin. Clarithromycin and azithromycin have advanced action against *Haemophilus influenzae* bacterium and lesser activity against MAC.

This class of drug can slow down bacterial growth and can be taken for either a few days to treat common bacterial infections such as nose and throat infections but can also be taken in the long term, for up to several years, to try and improve symptoms and reduce/ eliminate the number of infections.

A conservative approach is usually adopted and macrolides are usually prescribed for patients with more than two or three infections per year after they have used mucoactive drugs which are aimed at both reducing the amount of mucus produced in the lungs and helping to clear mucus from the lungs.

Macrolides can be used together with inhaled antibiotics for patients who continue to have more than two or three infections annually after taking long-term antibiotics. There were a number of options discussed in the European Respiratory Society (ERS) guidelines published in 2017, about treatments with macrolide and antibiotic drugs and whether inhalation or tablet form of antibiotic should be used.

Mucoactive medications

Mucoactive medications may have a direct impact on clearance of mucus from the airways. They have different methods of actions including;

- expectorants which promote the secretion of sputum, including those which aid and/or induce coughing
- mucolytics, such as carbocisteine, bromhexine hydrochloride or erdosteine, which thin mucus
- mucokinetics, which facilitate cough transportability (which counteracts ciliary transport impairment)
- mucoregulators, such as glucocorticosteroids (a class of steroidal hormones) which suppress the mechanisms underlying chronic mucus hypersecretion.

To date, bronchiectasis research has mainly focussed on mucolytics and mucokinetics/ expectorants [in the form of humidification, different concentrations of saline solutions, and mannitol (a diuretic)].

Anti-inflammatory therapies in bronchiectasis such as inhaled or oral corticosteroids have had few research findings and their positive bronchiectasis results have to be balanced against possible adverse side effects. It has been recommended by the British Thoracic Society (BTS) that they not be offered to patients unless there are other indicators such as chronic asthma, ABPA, COPD or inflammatory bowel disease.

Mucolytic drugs

If sputum is sticky and hard to cough up/ expel, a health care professional may suggest the use of a mucolytic drug, such as Carbocisteine, to break it up or the use of a nebuliser which contains the drug in the form of a saline salt solution, called a hypertonic saline, which can be inhaled.

A nebuliser will convert the liquid saline solution into a mist which can be breathed in; the process takes about ten minutes. As with most treatments, problems can be associated with taking an inhalation and the GP should be involved at all times. An inhaled treatment will normally initially last for 3-4 months and if it is successful it could be maintained long term.

Mucolytics may not be universally available.

Mucoregulators

Drugs that regulate mucus secretion or interfere with the DNA/F- actin (protein) network are mucregulatory agents. These include carbocisteine/ carbocysteine, anticholinergics, glucocorticoids and macrolide antibiotics.

Surgery

Treatment of bronchiectasis is usually started on a conservative basis with the use of medication, usually antibiotics, together with different forms of physiotherapy and possible lifestyle changes by the sufferer. If this approach is not successful and severe symptoms persist then surgery may be necessary. Before any surgery is carried out the patient's fitness is tested (CPET) and assessed.

Cardiopulmonary Exercise Testing (CPET)

CPET is an objective method of assessing patient fitness prior to surgery to guide patient care. It aims to improve postoperative outcomes, improve clinical efficiency and optimise patient's experience of the surgical journey. Fitness predicts postoperative complications and death. It is increasingly used by anaesthetists and perioperative (around the time of an operation) physicians and is available at many hospital trusts in the UK (the exact figure is not available). The CPET services in the UK doubled between 2011 and 2018 with 30,000 patients being seen annually. It is also being available abroad.

The physiology behind CPET, which is a stress test, examines the body's response to the increased intensity of exercise. It examines how the heart and lungs work and measures how oxygen consumption and carbon dioxide production take place and increases during the increased demands of planned levels of exercise. The testing equipment consists of a cycle ergometer, an ECG (electrocardiogram) and a mouth piece which analyses oxygen consumption and carbon dioxide production during changes of level of breathing.

After the testing and the results analysis, the patient (and family) will discuss the findings with a member of the team probably a Consultant Anaesthetist and possibilities will be discussed including the risk of mortality (death) and morbidity (changes in health); the possible alternatives to surgery; possible changes to medication; and perioperative care and postoperative location (level of ward care depending on level of risk).

Types of operation

If blood is continually coughed up (haemoptysis) during flare-ups, a pulmonary angiography (internal medical imaging) scan can look at the blood vessels in the lungs. If vessels are identified which are the cause of the bleeding then a procedure called embolisation which blocks off the affected blood vessels could be offered. Sometimes lung resection surgery can remove the area with abnormal vessels and associated bleeding.

Because any lung surgery is extremely serious and complicated, a multidisciplinary hospital team of respiratory specialists will decide on the options of lung resection or full transplant. They will take into account nutritional support and pre-operative pulmonary rehabilitation before surgical referral.

Lung surgery is carried out by a thoracic surgeon and can be one of the following;

- ❖ a wedge resection, when a piece of lung is removed
- ❖ a lobectomy, when an entire lobe of a lung is removed
- ❖ a pneumonectomy, when the entire lung is removed.

Lung transplantation is an established treatment for end-stage non-cystic fibrosis bronchiectasis. In fact, the combined UK transplant experience has suggested that bronchiectasis has one of the best post-transplant outcomes. Interestingly, it has been calculated that bronchiectasis has a better cost effectiveness outcome following lung transplant as compared to COPD, which is the most common indication for lung transplant.

Reports about the results of lung transplants

There is a dearth of published articles on this subject and there is a need for better data to assist international transplant centres and clinicians who treat patients with severe bronchiectasis. Published information, the references for which are found in the appendix, includes;

- ✓ a report by *Birch J et al.* which indicated that lung transplantation (carried out at the Freeman Hospital, Newcastle upon Tyne, England) is a useful therapeutic option for severe end-stage bronchiectasis and should be considered by physicians as an option for those with severe bronchiectasis. This has offered good lung transplant patient survival rates (74% survival @ year 1, 64% @ year 3, 61% @ year 5, and 48% @ year 10) and lung function outcomes. Its survival values were similar to other bilateral lung transplants which had been carried out
- ✓ a report from Germany by *Rademacher J et al.* reported good outcomes from bronchiectasis lung transplant patients. There was a survival rate of 83% in year one and 73% in year five
- ✓ a study by *Titman A et al.* studied lung transplantation between 1997 and 2006 for patients of bronchiectasis and other groups of lung conditions. Transplantation appeared to improve survival for all groups. It was also suggested that more work was required to inform better lung treatment allocation
- ✓ a study by *Nathan J A et al.* found that recipients with bronchiectasis and antibody deficiency had no worse prognosis than those with bronchiectasis alone.

Lung & airways clearance techniques and physiotherapy

Lung and airways clearance

The progressive damage and structural changes to airways in the lung(s) caused by bronchiectasis leads to an accumulation and pooling of stagnated and infected sputum in them. Natural defence mechanisms such as Mucociliary clearance (MCC) and cough mechanisms can't cope with this situation so gravity; breathing and physical exercises; and chest massage techniques are needed to clear the amassing secretions.

A simple and efficient way of clearing trapped secretions in the lung, by releasing and coughing them up, is to increase lung volume which results in an outward pull on the airway. This is achieved by deep breathing and exercise (exercise also speeds ciliary activity).

By clearing the sputum, antibiotics will be able to work better. Once a day bronchopulmonary therapy will lead to an improvement in cough symptoms and cough related health. At difficult times for a sufferer, regular twice daily physiotherapy will increase sputum expectoration (cough or spitting out phlegm/ sputum from the throat or lungs), improve cough-related health status, quality of life and exercise capacity.

Commonly, an airway clearance techniques session can last for between 10 and 30 minutes. At those times when an individual is very mucus productive, it is important that he/ she achieves a balance between maximising the clearance and not becoming fatigued or dizzy.

Every individual is different and this should be reflected in the session(s) length and intensity. They should meet the individual's needs and should probably be increased, if possible, during an infective exacerbation.

The patient can be taught suitable lung and airway clearance techniques by a specialised respiratory physiotherapist who will also educate the patient about their condition and give advice about exercise or inhaled/ oral therapy which may enhance the effectiveness of any airway clearance technique. Individuals using an airway clearance technique should be reviewed by a respiratory physiotherapist within three months of the initial appointment and this review should be part of any annual clinic appointment to ensure that the regimen is being optimised. Anyone with a condition deterioration should have their technique reviewed.

These airways clearance techniques include;

- ✓ postural drainage (PD) techniques which aim to encourage sputum to be drained away from the lungs while the patient is comfortably lying side down on the edge of a bed. Different positions can be tried to see which works best and the head should not be lower than the hips. Lying over a pillow or cushion could help. Sessions, depending

on the condition's severity, could be 1 – 3 times daily for a period of up to twenty minutes each
- ✓ physiotherapy - taught exercises for better breathing, especially the specific 'Active cycle of breathing techniques' (ACBT) (which in 2002 was taught by 91% of UK senior physiotherapists) and Autogenic drainage (AD).
- ✓ manual chest massage techniques (such as percussive chest clapping, vibrations and shaking) are used to loosen secretions, reduce stress and fatigue and assist other airways clearance techniques such as PD. Percussion in particular, can be done manually or by using a small, palm size electrical/ electronic muscle stimulator such as the excellent electronic iSmart massager (which I use) or a more common TENS machine.

A more detailed description of 'The Active cycle of breathing techniques' (ACBT) and 'Autogenic drainage' (AD) is given in chapter five.

Hydration and sputum clearance

Lack of hydration facilitates the build- up of thick secretions and it also impairs oxygen delivery. Fluid intake is a more effective expectorant in expelling sputum than an inhaled moisture which is largely utilised in the upper airways. It is therefore vital that a bronchiectasis sufferer maintains a sufficient fluid intake (possibly 6-8 glasses of water daily). The necessary amount will vary between individuals and their medical and other circumstances.

If fluid is inhaled it can either be steam, or in my case asafoetida vapour.

A patient can use any of a variety of available small devices which the patient can blow through in order to clear the chest of mucus. Some of these cause vibrations which loosen sputum and others open up the airways to help the sputum to move e.g. these devices include the acapella; flutter valve; and positive expiratory valve (PEP).

More details about the physiotherapy techniques which are aimed at clearing the airways and expelling mucus, ACBT and other techniques for the improvement of breathing are included in chapter five.

High frequency chest wall oscillation (HFCWO) therapy with the SmartVest Airway Clearance System and other similar devices

HFCWO is a therapy which was developed in the USA. The user wears an inflatable vest (which utilises air bladder technology) that is attached by hoses to an external generator and which delivers percussion to the chest wall through vibrations at high-frequency, Rapid and repeating pulses of positive air pressure (5-20 per second) gently oscillate (squeeze and release) the chest to loosen and thin mucus. After every few minutes, the user stops the machine and coughs or 'huffs' out the mucus (or has it suctioned out).

The 'huff' or 'huff coughing helps to move the mucus up from the lungs. The 'huff is in three parts (1) in-breath, (2) hold (3) active exhalation. The in-breath (1) and hold (2) allows air to get behind the mucus and separates it from the lung wall so it can be coughed out/ expectorated (3).

The HFCWO treatment encompasses percussive (tapping) chest massage and postural airways clearance. This is easier to achieve with the machine doing the work but has the same goal – clearance of mucus. It is tailored to the individual and usually a session lasts for about thirty minutes; starting with low pressures and frequencies that increase until a recommended pressure and frequency is reached. It is carried out in the sitting position but this can be adjusted to allow for mobility if standing or when lying down.

HFCWO has been used as a component of mucus clearance for people suffering from cystic fibrosis and studies have been conducted to investigate its use for treating bronchiectasis. The results of the study by *Powner J. & NeSmith A. et al. 'Employment of an Algorithm of Care including Chest Physiotherapy Reduced Hospitalizations and Stability of Lung Function in Bronchiectasis'* was published in the journal *BMC Pulmonary Medicine 19, Article number:82 (2019) 25.4.*

This was the first long-term study which involved a treatment algorithm for bronchiectasis that involved standard therapies and standardised chest physiotherapy with HFCWO. Based on its results, the research team from the University of Alabama, USA concluded that a care regimen involving HFCWO 'may help to reduce the decline in lung function, the need for oral antibiotics and the hospitalisation rate'. The algorithm was also associated with reduced exacerbations. All the categories of improvements had financial and quality of life implications.

In the UK, different NHS Trusts make provision to supply a HFCWO device and other airway clearance device to children and young people (CYP) on either a sale or rental basis. There are large variations in how equipment is funded across services in England, Scotland and Wales. These variations may depend on local Clinical Commissioning Group (CCG) agreements. It is worth making enquiries with your local Trust or CCG about the position in your locality whether you are an adult or have responsibility for a child or young person (CYP). As at February 2020 in Australia there was no evidence for the use of this type of device for children with non-CF bronchiectasis.

For the readers' information, the American company which manufactures the Smart Vest system which was worn by participants in the study was Electromed. This device can now be managed using an app on either a smartphone or tablet via Bluetooth technology. Another American manufacturer is Hillrom Services which makes and supplies the 'Vest'.

Airway clearance using a Mechanical in/exsufflation (MI-E) device

An MI-E device, is a portable cough assist device (CAD) machine, which is used to help clear an airway of mucus when a person is unable to do this satisfactorily him/herself. These devices are especially valuable for people who suffer from neuromuscular diseases or spinal cord injuries where muscle weakness may inhibit the ability to cough.

The machine provides a quick positive pressure followed by a quick negative pressure. With the positive pressure, the lungs expand with air (insufflation) and then expel the air with negative pressure (exsufflation). The repeated cycle of alternating positive and negative pressure stimulates an artificial cough. The cycles are repeated until a person doesn't expel any more secretions.

The MI-E device can be seen as an alternative or adjunct to other ventilating and clearance methods such as suction, intermittent positive pulmonary ventilation (IPPV), handheld flutter valve, acapella device or cornet device. Whilst the MI-E device is more expensive than the aforementioned alternatives it does have a number of advantages such as requiring less work and being more comfortable.

Some MI-E devices have additional features. The 'Nippy Clearway' for example as well as being MI-E also includes Intermittent Positive Pressure Breathing (IPPB), Non-Invasive Ventilator (NIV) and Oscillation Mode features.

Instructional videos available on the internet

The Australian health organisation 'Bronchiectasis Toolbox' (see www.bronchiectasis.com.au) has produced a number of excellent, simple instructional videos on its website which deal with a number of ways breathing dysfunction can be addressed and improved. These videos are aimed amongst other things at improving lung ventilation, helping the clearance of excess secretions and the improved function of the diaphragm and pelvic floor muscles. They also stress the importance of the patient and therapist (or family helper) interacting with each other and working as a team. The videos cover;

- the Active cycle of breathing technique (ACBT)
- the Forced Expiration Technique
- Positive Expiratory Pressure Therapy using 'Pari PEP' or 'mask PEP' or 'Thera PEP'
- Oscillating Positive Expiratory Pressure Therapy using 'Acapella' or 'Bottle PEP' or a 'PARi O-PEP'
- autogenic drainage and manual techniques
- nebuliser therapy
- breathing dysfunction.

Pulmonary rehabilitation /respiratory rehabilitation programmes (PR)

Pulmonary Rehabilitation (PR) is an exercise and education programme for people with long-term lung disease, including bronchiectasis, who experience breathlessness and who want to better understand

and manage their condition and its symptoms. It is also recommended for people leaving hospital after a COPD flare-up.

While some people may not be suitable for the programme (after a discussion with the GP), as there is a waiting lists in some areas it is a great idea for possible candidates to see about attending as soon as possible.

After completing a PR programme, participants will have learnt and experienced how to exercise safely at the right level; meet others in a similar health situation; and have fun. For the programme to really work fully, the participant has to be committed to attend the full course and follow the advice which has been given by the team.

The Pulmonary Rehabilitation (PR) programme

Its importance is such that the UK National Health System (NHS) has included (section 3) pulmonary rehabilitation as a key intervention in its 2019 Long Term Plan (www.longtermplan.nhs.uk), for the next ten years, which has made respiratory disease a new national clinical priority. See the BTS comments on pages 28/29.

Those bronchiectasis and other respiratory conditions (mainly COPD and pulmonary fibrosis) sufferers who experience the symptom of severe shortage of breath can be referred by a GP, practice nurse or hospital respiratory team to a PR programme which is held on an out- patient basis at a local hospital or other venue. A list of hospitals offering specialist bronchiectasis services in Scotland, England and Northern Ireland can be found on page 5 of the website: www.bronchiectasishelp.org.uk

The programme can either be on an outpatient basis, an inpatient basis or home-based. Each of these settings have advantages and disadvantages. If the programme is held in a group setting, it is over a 6 – 8 weeks period with 2 sessions weekly of two hours each.

The programme while not being able to reverse lung damage is aimed to help a sufferer benefit from the modifications to the disability that comes from it. It aims to help participants;

- ✓ become more physically active e.g. increase muscle strength, so oxygen is used more efficiently
- ✓ cough less
- ✓ cope better with feeling out of breath (dyspnoea)
- ✓ improve fitness, so confidence to do everyday tasks increases e.g. walking further, climbing stairs, going shopping etc
- ✓ feel generally better physically and mentally and have a better quality of life
- ✓ be less likely to have chest infections/ exacerbations
- ✓ have a reduction in number of acute and emergency hospital admissions and GP appointments
- ✓ return to work

✓ reduce financial and time expenditure associated with GP and hospital visits.

An initial individualised health and abilities assessment could include any of the following - the 6-minute walk test (MWT), the incremental paced shuttle walking test (ISWT) or a stair climbing exercise.

Following this initial assessment, each of the programme's sessions will, for half the time, comprise specialised physical exercises including aerobic exercise and resistance training which is again tailored to the individual's capabilities. The rest of the time is spent taking in information about looking after the body, and the lungs in particular; advice on ways of managing the condition such as how to eat healthily; how to maximise night-time sleep; what to do when you are unwell and how to manage anxiety/stress; and cope with cough incontinence. Participant socialising is an important element in the programme.

The supervising team are trained health professionals; usually including a physiotherapist, exercise physiologist, nurse, dietician and occupational therapist.

Cough incontinence

Bladder leakage (urinary incontinence) can be associated with long-term coughing, due to the extra pressure it puts on the pelvis and pelvic floor muscles. This can be addressed by following a personalised treatment plan which is devised with the guidance of a respiratory physiotherapist. Depending on the results of a continence assessment, the plan can include pelvic floor strengthening, urge - suppression techniques, bladder emptying voiding techniques and bladder re-training. Please also see page 258.

Healthy eating and drinking

The importance of eating healthily and drinking the correct amount of water cannot be underestimated for general and bladder health. Not only will this help the body fight infections but mucous can be thinned which should help it be expelled.

The use of inspiratory muscle training as an adjunct to conventional pulmonary rehabilitation can be considered as this should enhance the maintenance of the positive results of the PR programme.

More details about healthy lifestyle including exercise, diet and sleeping are contained in chapter six.

After attending the Pulmonary Rehabilitation (PR) programme

To maintain the health and everyday living improvements gained by completing the Pulmonary Rehabilitation (PR) programme it is important for the participant(s) to continue putting into practice the positive principles which have been learnt on the course. Interestingly, in the *ERS Guidelines on adult bronchiectasis (published in 2017)* it was concluded that the benefits of PR achieved in 6 to 8 weeks are maintained for 3 to 6 months. A way to extend this period is to undertake a suitable exercise activity which they enjoy. Some participants, if they prefer, can also be referred to an organised exercise course as a follow up to the structured PR programme. The PR team will be pleased to advise about availability, suitability and cost of these exercise courses.

If someone's good work having attended the PR programme is lost, then for them it is likely that there will be;

- an increase in breathlessness, even when doing simple tasks
- a decrease in fitness, with jobs not being finished
- more exacerbations and visits to the GP and hospital
- a deterioration in their quality of life, with associated isolation and depression.

Home Exercise Programmes (HEP)

Sometimes, because of time restraints and financial limitations, a suitable candidate will not be able to attend a PR programme. If this is the case, they can follow a Home Exercise Programme (HEP) as an alternative. The HEP can also be used by those who have completed a PR programme and who would prefer to continue to exercise at home rather than going to an outside venue (especially in the dark, cold months of winter when cold air can be detrimental to breathing and the lungs).

It is a positive step to try to keep a daily HEP activity diary to see how progress is being made over time. While this diary is relatively easy to design there are number of internet sites which describe PR and HEP and contain blank model exercise result sheets.

An excellent, helpful example, is the information leaflet No. IL411, author *Cowan H*, which has been produced by the respiratory physiotherapy department of the Queen Elizabeth Hospital, Gateshead, England entitled *'Pulmonary Rehabilitation, Home Exercise Programme, Cardio/Respiratory Physiotherapy Team'* (www.qegateshead.nhs.uk).

The diary entry notes may be helpful to the GP or consultant when a patient has to visit either/ both of them.

Helping breathing and reducing breathlessness

Helping breathing

The following actions may further help people's breathing, especially those who suffer from breathlessness;

- ✓ the out- breath should be longer than the in-breath – this will allow the lungs time to empty and so encourage the lungs to fill up fully on the next breath

- ✓ try to slow down the speed of breathing – in through the nose; and out through the mouth. This should reduce coughing, gives the lungs more time to fill with air and boost direct nitric oxide delivery to the lungs
- ✓ try to maintain a good posture, with no slouching when standing or sitting – this will allow the lungs to empty/ fill more easily and reduce bodily pressure on them
- ✓ remember, if appropriate, to use a nebuliser or inhaler properly to help keep the airways open
- ✓ increase airflow towards your face by opening a window or using a fan.

More information about improving breathing is contained in chapter five.

Reducing breathlessness

People with lung conditions, including bronchiectasis, often get tired and/ or short of breath (dyspnoea) when doing everyday tasks in and around the house as well as when carrying out exercises such as walking, gardening, running, cycling or swimming.

It is very important to conserve as much energy as possible to enable activities to be completed and have some left over for exercise purposes which should improve the quality of someone's health. Whilst a respiratory physiotherapist or occupational therapist can offer advice on this subject, the following points could be considered by a sufferer to make their life easier and more bearable;

- ✓ breathing exercises can be learnt and practised to help breathing be done more efficiently and with less effort and stress on the respiratory system and the body
- ✓ rests can be taken between tasks and these should be done in a position where posture is good with pressure on the lungs and stomach being minimised
- ✓ jobs can be planned ahead, with necessary tools or utensils being gathered together before starting the activity (which can be broken down and done in its component parts)
- ✓ work at a steady pace and don't go mad at one time and then be lethargic the next
- ✓ good body mechanics such as lifting with a straight back with bent knees with the object close to the body and with twisting movements being avoided should all help minimise effort
- ✓ try to sit down when doing activities; minimise arm movements and avoid bending/ reaching/ twisting. Long handled, and other, aids can help pick up objects from the floor and a towelling robe can replace a towel when drying oneself
- ✓ if possible, consider moving from a house to a flat which is serviced by a reliable lift or to a bungalow or other similar type of property with only a ground floor. Alternatively, consider installing an electrically powered stair lift in your house – this will obviate the tiring need to climb stairs and it

can be used to carry objects such as a washing basket full of clean/ dirty clothes.

A self-management treatment programme

While there is a great input into the treatment of bronchiectasis by the medical profession – GP, hospital consultants, respiratory physiotherapists, dieticians, nurses and other specialists, the individual needs to take responsibility for improving their own well- being with actions they can take. These actions can include;

- ✓ keeping your lungs clear, as much as possible, following the advice of a respiratory physiotherapist and also taking into account your own efforts
- ✓ keeping as active as possible and doing appropriate physical and flexibility exercises which preferably should be fun for you and which can be done with simple equipment
- ✓ breathe correctly – in through the nose and exhale from an open mouth
- ✓ when necessary, taking medicines or using inhalers as prescribed and not letting them run out. A reserve can be kept in case of a flare-up
- ✓ knowing how much sputum is normally produced and its colour/ consistency
- ✓ submitting a sputum sample at least once a year and have a prepared flare-up plan
- ✓ having an annual check with your GP
- ✓ getting a flu, and any other advised, inoculation jab annually

- ✓ not seeing anyone who is unwell with a cold, flu or chest infection (especially sickly young children who seem to distribute their germs at will!)
- ✓ improving your breathing technique
- ✓ **if a smoker – give up, especially if pregnant or are around babies and small children as it can badly affect their health through passive smoking!!!** Much advice and help about quitting is available from the GP or pharmacy for you
- ✓ drinking lots of fluid and eating healthily. Keep to recommended alcohol limits
- ✓ trying to keep your weight under control and, if it gives you concerns or you think that it is excessive, talk to your GP who can explain your options such as referring you to a dietitian or slimming club
- ✓ staying socially active and talk to a family member, friend or colleague about your bronchiectasis and how it affects you
- ✓ considering joining a local breathing support group or club – the GP practice will have details
- ✓ when sleeping, experiment to see if different lying positions help. Side-lying has been shown to have advantages in helping the lungs and breathing become more efficient
- ✓ try different breathing methods. It is more economical to increase breathing through breathing deeper rather than faster
- ✓ taking vitamin B which can mitigate damage done by exposure to fine particle pollution
- ✓ having a good intake of vitamin D – found in salmon tuna and other oily fish, evaporated milk,

white meats and other food sources (many informative websites); in supplements; and in sunlight (to get UVB); this will help the immune system and reduce colonisation by bacteria which can be the cause of inflammation flare-ups, more hospital visits and poorer health- related quality of life
- ✓ using eco-friendly air fresheners and clothes washing detergents
- ✓ keeping the workplace or home free from dust and other irritants
- ✓ trying to avoid traffic pollution
- ✓ if breathing problems are caused by exposure to certain plants and crops try to avoid them and any associated pesticides or fungicides
- ✓ considering using a dry salt inhaler which is drug free and designed to draw excess fluid from the sinuses, cleanse the respiratory system and open the airways to encourage better breathing.

The detrimental effects of air pollution on respiratory conditions was highlighted in the report '*Acute Effects of Air Pollution on Hospital Admissions for Asthma, COPD and Bronchiectasis in Ahvaz, Iran*' by Raji H et al, published on 3 March 2020 in *Int Journ of Chronic Obstructive Pul Disease Vol 15, pages 501-514.* This report found that short-term exposure to air pollutants significantly increases the risk of hospital admissions for these three conditions in the adult and elderly population in this city.

Differences between children's and adult's bronchiectasis

While children's bronchiectasis is similar to that in adults, there are also large differences. The main differences relate to the extent of clinical symptoms; radiological diagnosis; criteria and prognosis. It is important that all children with bronchiectasis are investigated to ascertain the underlying cause.

Congenital (present from birth) bronchiectasis only affects young children whereas non-congenital bronchiectasis typically affects adults and older children.

Children's airway damage is superimposed upon the physiological changes associated with lung growth and development. Importantly with children, there is an opportunity to diagnose and manage bronchiectasis early and this will influence outcomes.

Research in 2010 by *Chang A B et al. 'Bronchiectasis and suppurative lung disease in children and adults in Australia and New Zealand'* pub *Med. J.Aust 193: 356 -365* indicated that 80% of non- smoking adults who were newly diagnosed had symptoms since childhood and that the duration of chronic cough which is the most common symptom is related to lung function at the time of diagnosis. How these comments ring true to the author!

Children with bronchiectasis don't necessarily have a persistent cough but rather an intermittent chronic cough. Because they have a limited ability to discharge/ expectorate airway mucus/ phlegm secretions the term 'productive' cough is used instead of 'wet' cough particularly with young children. The duration of the chronic cough relates to the condition's severity as shown on the chest HRCT scan.

When diagnosed early, children's bronchiectasis is mainly the cylindrical/ tubular subtype. Unlike in adults, pseudomonas (bacteria) infection is rare.

As there are limitations and small cancer risks in children's (c)HRCT radiological (chest high resolution computed tomography) scans the term chronic suppurative lung disease (CSLD) is used to describe a diagnosis where there are clinical symptoms without a HRCT confirmation.

Causes of children's bronchiectasis

Children's bronchiectasis causes include;

- a severe viral or bacterial respiratory tract infection e.g. pneumonia, TB or whooping cough
- an immune system/ immune deficiency problem which leads to probably more bacterial infections
- a lung development problem, such as being born premature with the lungs being too small and underdeveloped so more likely to get an infection
- a blockage caused by the inhalation of a small object such as a pea
- an underlying inherited genetic disease such as cystic fibrosis (CF) (which is caused by a single specific genetic problem) or primary ciliary

dyskinesia (PCD). Other conditions, including asthma, are caused by a combination of a number of genetic and environmental factors such as air pollution
- accidental breathing - in stomach acid that has come up via the oesophagus
- CVS (cyclical vomiting syndrome) or an underlying inflammatory bowel disease could give abdominal pain or diarrhoea which may suggest a secondary bronchiectasis
- Infections, such as meningitis in non-respiratory organ systems, may suggest underlying immune deficiencies.

An excellent organisation in Australia which considers all aspects about how bronchiectasis can affect both adults and children, and details about methods by which it can be treated and managed is 'Bronchiectasis Toolbox' (www.bronchiectasis.com.au). This organisation's work is supported by the Australian Physiotherapy Association, Lung Foundation Australia, Institute for Breathing and Sleep, and the Alfred (Health).

A good summary information sheet about bronchiectasis (*www.kidshealth.org.nz/bronchiectasis*) which is aimed at children (and their family) has been produced by the kidshealth organisation in New Zealand *(www.kidshealth.org.nz)*.

Symptoms of children's bronchiectasis

Children's bronchiectasis symptoms include;

- a persistent cough, especially between colds and infections, that produces a lot of mucus
- mucus may contain blood when it is coughed up
- feeling very tired or possibly wheezing when they breathe. More breathless than expected after exercising -wheezing or crackling noises may be heard
- mucus is hard to digest and it may be vomited up if it has been swallowed
- if diagnosis of asthma has been made and it hasn't got better with treatment or there are lots of chest infections with yellow/ green mucus they may have bronchiectasis
- 'clubbing' of the child's fingers or toes when there is a loss of angle between the nail and nail bed and if well developed a bulbous end to the digits. It shows fluid accumulation and is possibly linked to protein levels.

Diagnosis of children's bronchiectasis

It is vital for people of all ages who demonstrate the clinical symptoms of bronchiectasis, or other respiratory condition, to be diagnosed as soon as possible so that the appropriate treatment can be applied speedily. This is especially so in the case of children and young people.

Triggers for referral to a specialist by the GP include - two or more episodes of a chronic productive/ wet cough lasting more than 4 weeks which respond to antibiotics and a chest radiograph abnormality lasting for more than 6 weeks after an appropriate treatment.

A family medical history is taken similar to that with an adult with suspected bronchiectasis. This will identify whether family members have similar symptoms and whether the child has been exposed to tobacco smoke at home by experiencing 'passive smoking'.

Details of symptoms soon after birth should be taken to identify causes due to congenital abnormalities such as immune deficiencies e.g. CF (cystic fibrosis) or PCD (primary ciliary dyskinesia). These can be compared with those which occur at a later date e.g. after inhaling a foreign body or acute infections e.g. influenza.

The tests for child bronchiectasis diagnosis are very similar to those for adults but do vary slightly. The tests include;

- using a HRCT chest scan to see if the airways are widened. This will give a more detailed assessment of structural lung damage than a plain chest X-ray. A low dose CT scan should be used, as adequate images can be produced at a fraction of radiation which is important for children
- checking a cough, especially if it has lasted daily for more than four weeks which is not normal and if it is present with other problems such as chest wheezing or breathing fast when being active

- testing the mucus to find out if bacteria are present and if so, which type. An annual sputum sample screening could be considered for those who are able to expectorate (cough or spitting up sputum to clear lungs)
- after about 6 years of age children should be able to perform meaningful and repeatable spirometry tests which will give details about lung function. Under 6 years, useful spirometry is unlikely to be performed and results of alternative tests are unreliable. Lung function tests may also include lung volume tests
- other complex pulmonary-function tests and the 6-minute walk test are sometimes used to determine functional impairment. Objective tests will provide information about disease severity and its prognosis
- taking blood tests to check the immune system
- using a small bronchoscope camera on the end of a tube to look into the lungs
- checking sweat to see if they have cystic fibrosis
- testing to see if there is gastro-oesophageal acid reflux up from the stomach
- checking for small inhaled foreign bodies such as a pea or small toy e.g. a piece of lego
- checking to see if the hair-like structures on the respiratory tract's cilia cells are working properly; this is a test for primary ciliary dyskinesia (PCD)and is most appropriate for older children.

Very helpful and informative advice about children's coughing and respiratory health can be found in the leaflet *'Cough in Children'* which is published on the KidsHealth NZ website *(www.kidshealth.org.nz/cough-children).*

Children's bronchiectasis examination

A child's examination for suspected bronchiectasis should include;

- ❖ overall growth parameters and comparison to age - matched normal values as some cause of the condition can directly influence growth
- ❖ resting respiratory rate and associated respiratory signs e.g. cough, shallow breathing and wheeze and increased rate of breathing when exerted
- ❖ craniofacial abnormalities and neurological degenerative conditions which may explain underlying bronchiectasis
- ❖ digital clubbing which may indicate length of time of bronchiectasis
- ❖ chest examination which should include an assessment of thoracic expansion
- ❖ listening (auscultation) to sounds from the lungs.

Because bronchiectasis is a progressive condition, the key to treating it effectively for children and young people (and adults) is early diagnosis.

Treatments of children's bronchiectasis

Earlier in this chapter the aims of the treatment of bronchiectasis were listed and it is worth reiterating them at this stage. They are;

- ✓ preventing and suppressing acute and chronic bronchial infections
- ✓ preventing mucus clogging up the airway and so reducing airflow
- ✓ controlling and improving the condition's symptoms such as coughing up/ clearing mucus and tiredness
- ✓ reducing chest infection(s) and flare-ups
- ✓ preventing further progressive lung damage and reducing the impact of structural lung disease
- ✓ reducing complications such as reduced lung function and coughing up blood
- ✓ improving the sufferer's quality of life by making the condition easier to live with
- ✓ achieving a balance between the potential beneficial effects of intervention against the burden of treatment and the risk of adverse effects from it.

The treatments for children's (and young persons) bronchiectasis are broadly similar to those of adults but obviously there have to be adjustments made because of their younger age. It is imperative that mucus from the damaged areas of the lung is reduced and that airways clearance is maximised. As with adults, the management of bronchiectasis should be by a multidisciplinary team; the input from members of the family should not be underestimated and encouraged.

It is important that bronchiectasis is diagnosed early and children receive optimal treatment because some studies have shown that when this happens, lung function can stabilise and improve over the next five years. Other studies have shown that early radiologically- diagnosed bronchiectasis is reversible. (sources: article by *Nelson S W and Christoforidis 'Reversible Bronchiectasis' pub in RSNA 'Radiology' journal Vol 71, no. 3* and report by *Kucuk C, Turkkani M H & Arda K 'A case report of reversible bronchiectasis in an adult: Pseudobronchiestasis' published in Res Med Case reports, Vol 26, 2019 pages 315-316)*

Worryingly, a study in Australia has suggested that children with bronchiectasis have poorer lung function than those with cystic fibrosis when comparing the different levels of care, using several criteria, given to children with these conditions and are deserving of improved multidisciplinary care. This study by *Prentice B.J. et al, 'Children with bronchiectasis have poorer lung function than those with cystic fibrosis and do not receive the same standard of care'* was published in the journal *Paediatric Pulmonology. Vol 54, Issue 12, pages 1867-2053 Dec 2019 (online 1.9.2019).*

The forms of treatment for paediatric bronchiectasis mainly consist of;

- medication, especially antibiotics at a low dose to treat and hopefully prevent frequent flare-ups/ exacerbations

- taking a bronchodilator medication to help relax muscles in the chest and clear the airways by using a handheld inhaler, tablets, syrup or by nebuliser
- different chest physiotherapy techniques including tapping (percussion) on the chest; using devices to be blown into and improved breathing system exercises
- keeping children active by doing exercises such as trampolining which will help to clear mucus
- having a healthy diet and drinking enough to help fight infections and thin mucus
- prevention, which includes the reduced exposure to smoke (especially direct and passive tobacco smoking/vaping) and others' infections.

Child patients should have an updated overall action plan provided for them after each outpatient appointment which should include a plan for when they are well and also a plan for when they are unwell.

The KidsHealth NZ organisation (www.kidshealth.org.uk) has produced a good bronchiectasis information sheet for schools which includes advice about the importance of exercise and good lifestyle (www.kidshealth.org.nz/bronchiectasis-information-schools).

Emergency advice for children's treatment

Although bronchiectasis is usually treated in a routine way at home under the guidance of a GP and/ or consultant, if a bad infection happens then there may be need for an admission to hospital for treatment including intensive respiratory physiotherapy.

It is necessary to get help immediately by phoning the emergency ambulance service (phone 999 in the UK) if any of the following apply;

- **the child's skin turns pale or blue or their tongue and lips are blue**
- **the child is struggling to breathe or is breathing faster than usual and there are shorter regular pauses in their breathing when they are awake**
- **the child's breathing stops for more than 20 seconds on any occasion**
- **the child is unable to wake up, or when woken is very drowsy and doesn't stay awake**
- **the child's temperature is above 38°C (101°F)**
- **the child is coughing up blood**
- **the child is making a grunting noise when breathing out**
- **the child has had a fit or is having a fit and this has never happened before**
- **the medicine the child is taking is not making him/ her better.**

Medication for the different causes of children's bronchiectasis.

Antibiotic drugs is the main form of medication and after discussion with the doctor it will be decided if they are to be taken orally. The prescribing should be based on regular assessment of airway microbiology. If the patient is more poorly, then a hospital admission may be necessary and the antibiotics will be administered intravenously directly into the bloodstream through a drip.

Antibiotics may be directed directly into the airways in mist form, through a nebuliser in most cases. if there are problems in moving the mucus and clearing the airways a nebuliser may also be used to deliver a hypertonic salt water solution into the lungs. The GP/consultant will discuss with the family the benefits and risks, including future antibiotic resistance, of taking antibiotics.

If cystic fibrosis (CF) is the cause, children may benefit from different medicines than those which are prescribed for non- cystic fibrosis bronchiectasis (NCFBE).

Macrolide therapy may be beneficial as it is aimed at direct anti-inflammatory action rather than antimicrobial action. It can be taken either daily or three times a week.

Children should have regular flu and other vaccinations as recommended. The multidisciplinary team members looking after the child's treatment will advise on the use of medications such as bronchodilators; corticosteroids; mucolytic agents and macrolide therapy.

Surgery for children

Surgery may be considered for child patients;

- ✓ when localised disease has not responded to other treatment
- ✓ when an obstructing tumour or foreign body needs removing
- ✓ when massive bleeding indicates a bronchial artery embolism
- ✓ when in severe cases a lung transplant may be required.

The physiotherapy assessment

Because children and young people are developing and changing physically, intellectually and emotionally, any physical assessment made by the therapist has to take into account behavioural and psychosocial issues which arise.

It is essential for parents or care givers to be involved in the communication process with the child to help the child's confidence and cooperation. The parent can give the therapist important feedback about what works and what doesn't. Adolescents (12-18 years), should be encouraged to be open and independent in their views, this will help enable optimal and individualised treatment regimes.

At the initial assessment and during subsequent treatment sessions the therapist should listen to the child's actual comments and the nature of the cough and observe 'body language' in respect of things such as the cough itself, posture, activity and breathing levels. The assessment categories will be similar to those of adults and will include;

- what is usual (the baseline) especially the cough's frequency/ sound/ pattern etc
- the history of the respiratory illness
- the cough and sputum (thickness, colour etc)
- exercise & activity levels
- airway clearance techniques and inhalation & breathing techniques being used
- medications being taken
- results of X-rays and images/ scans
- assessment of the musculoskeletal condition
- stress incontinence if any.

The use of physiotherapy in paediatric bronchiectasis combines expert clinical experience and moderate evidence- based information. It is important that the treatment programme is reviewed regularly to ensure that airway clearance is being done correctly, to overcome any difficulties and to ensure that the treatment is being optimised. There should be full communication between the therapist and patient (and family support) while treatment is ongoing.

Airway Clearance Techniques (ACT)

Respiratory physiotherapy plays an important and established part in managing bronchiectasis because it helps move and clear secretions from the airways. The respiratory (physio)therapist will recommend the most appropriate type of physiotherapy taking into account the child's age and the severity of the bronchiectasis and its symptoms. Different techniques might be suitable for different age groups i.e. infants (0-1 years), toddlers (1-3), children (4-12) and adolescents (12-18).

To help move and clear airways secretions the therapist might recommend any of the following; an aiding device for the child to blow into; specific breathing exercises; moving the child into different positions while doing finger tapping percussions on their chest.

To make the clearance of mucus easier, the therapist might use a nebulised salt water solution before a session. It may however be difficult to persuade infants and young children to wear a nebuliser mask and distraction techniques may be necessary to allow this to happen.

In addition, young people can be distracted by having something else like TV or music playing while doing the clearance. It should, as far as possible, become an enjoyable part of their routine rather than a chore to be avoided.

A useful guide to appropriate airway clearance techniques for children and young people in the different age categories (see above for definitions) is included in the website
www.bronchiectasis.com.au/paediatrics/airway-clearance/choosing-the-correct-technique

Staying active

Regular, balanced exercise is important for maintaining and improving overall health as well as helping to clear the lungs of excess mucus. It should be done several times weekly and a structured and adaptable programme should bring many health benefits including aiding sputum clearance.

Exercise should include;

- ✓ cardiovascular and endurance training
- ✓ muscle strengthening
- ✓ balance, mobility and flexibility exercises.

Many children with mild bronchiectasis may have little activity limitation and should be able to take part in vigorous sports and games. Obviously, the types of children's activity and exercise will depend on their age and capabilities.

Toddlers and young children should have a fun element incorporated in their activities during a physiotherapy session and elsewhere. The physical element (e.g. soccer or trampolining) can be mixed with other techniques (e.g. percussive chest tapping) to help mucus clearance.

Exercises can be carried out in different positions where the effects of gravity on ventilation can be utilised. A treatment session should always end with physical activity or thoracic expansion exercises so that the airways remain as open as possible.

Exercise should be varied without strain being placed on the developing body. Weight bearing exercises such as swimming and trampolining being mixed in for example with football and tennis.

Alternative exercises can replace existing ones to reduce boredom and routine setting in. Expensive equipment and large spaces are not needed and weather needs to be considered so that if it rains or snows children can move indoors. If the weather outside is cold it is not advisable to do exercises which stimulate deep breathing.

Sufficient water should be drunk to avoid dehydration and appropriate footwear and clothing should be worn. The warm- up and cool- down should be part of an activity session.

Bronchodilators and supplemental oxygen should be available and used if necessary. Breathing games can be part of a session – this could be the case for children and adults without breathing problems as well. These games should have a fun element.

Most activities, especially in a group/ class setting can be social by encouraging interaction with others.

Weight bearing exercise increases bone mineral density.

Some exercises such as cycling and walking in town carry risks which have to be considered and safety clothing and helmets may need to be worn. It is more important for the parent to know how much activity is appropriate for the child than to follow generalised guidelines.

If the child is not interested in playing sports, they could be encouraged to sing or play a wind or brass instrument and both activities should help develop their lungs and breathing capabilities.

If computer games are the centre of someone's interest, the player could be encouraged to simulate in real life some of the exercises, such as running and jumping, which are shown on the screen by their superhero or heroine.

It is also important that children see adults enjoying being active.

Two excellent photo descriptions of physiotherapy exercises for very young and young children with chronic respiratory conditions can be found in the Paediatrics exercise section of the Bronchiectasis Toolbox website (www.bronchiectasis.com.au/paediatrics/physiotherapy/exercise). With suitable adjustments, the exercises shown could also be used by children without respiratory conditions.

Healthy diet and drinking enough

If a child (or adult) is continually coughing and fighting off infections this uses up energy and more healthy food is needed to cater for this. The immune system must be maintained especially by proteins and vitamins. Vitamin D, which is important for the immune system as well as for other body functions, is especially significant because some bronchiectasis sufferers are deficient in this. Vitamin D is naturally obtained from sunlight (UVB rays); from oily fish such as tuna, salmon and mackerel and many other food sources (information can be found by accessing the internet or by consulting a dietician/ nutritionist); or by taking vitamin supplements.

Drinking water (and not sugary or energy drinks) and soups help to keep mucus thin and easier to expel through coughing.

Children should be allowed to cough when they need to as it is paramount that their mucus is cleared. They should not be embarrassed to cough and if others get annoyed by this, the situation should be politely explained to them.

Prevention during pregnancy

Important risk factors that make the baby's (previously foetus) lung problems more likely is either a premature birth or low birth weight. It is most important that the pregnant mother and those around her lead as healthy a life as possible in order that the baby is able to benefit. Exposure to tobacco smoke and air pollution, with their particulate matter, is more likely to make a premature birth more likely and a possible likelihood of a linked baby's reduced lung development.

Following a healthy diet during the mother's pregnancy will reduce the risk of a low birth weight (less than 2.5 kg/ 5lbs 8 ozs) and the risk of symptoms such as wheezing, asthma and respiratory infections throughout the child's life. The NHS has a website 'eating a healthy diet in pregnancy' which gives a lot of useful information.

Flare-ups/ exacerbations/ chest infections

There are several ways that the risk of a flare- up/ exacerbation/ chest infection can be minimised or prevented. These include;

- ✓ not allowing the child or anyone around them i.e. family and friends to smoke and use tobacco products and e-cigarettes. The effects of direct or passive smoking can damage the lungs and throat, increase the chance of contracting an infection and make the infection's symptoms worse. Smoking

during pregnancy should be avoided and as early exposure to smoke can damage the lungs perhaps legislation should be introduced against smoking anywhere around children
- ✓ it is important to keep the flu jab and other vaccinations up to date. Sometimes it may be necessary to explain to a nurse or other medical practitioner that regular antibiotics are being taken for the treatment of bronchiectasis
- ✓ if a child is coughing more than usual, or if there is more/ differently coloured mucus than usual, a doctor should be contacted as soon as possible so that any treatment can start without delay
- ✓ to reduce the risk of a flare-up being triggered, a child should not be exposed to other people's colds and other infections. Obviously, there are difficulties in achieving this, at school or in the nursery or their social club environment, as many children seem always to be messengers for the various viruses that are generally going about
- ✓ always try to keep the home, especially the child's bedding, as clean as possible to reduce the risk of pollution being the cause of a flare-up.
- ✓ try not to go to polluted areas unless it is necessary and avoid busy roads and junctions where traffic air pollution is highest. A face protective mask/ covering could be worn.

Children's care action plan

All children and young people who have been diagnosed with bronchiectasis should be given a care action plan that assists them and their parents with their self-management if they are – well; unwell but able to attend a crèche or school; or unwell and not able to attend a crèche or school.

A clear example of this type of care action plan will be found at www.bronchiectasis.com.au/wp-content/uploads/2015/09/Paediatrics-Physiotherapy-Care-Plan.pdf.

Organs and Parts of the Body Which Affect Respiration

What is Respiration?

Respiration is the process whereby oxygen gas is inhaled (breathed in) from the surrounding air and transferred to the bloodstream and then transported around the body. Waste material in the form of carbon dioxide is expelled by the action of exhaling (breathing out). This process is known as the Gas Exchange.

Breathing is controlled by the respiratory centre in the brainstem. No conscious effort is needed to inhale and exhale air but the depth of breathing can be altered voluntarily.

During vigorous exercise, the heart and other muscles will need more oxygen and the breathing rate will increase accordingly. An adult at rest will breathe between 13 and 17 times per minute, this could increase to 80 breaths during exercise (these figures vary between people). Even at maximum exercise intensity only 70% of possible lung capacity is used. In contrast, a newborn baby will usually breathe at 40 breaths per minute and their deep breaths will be from the abdomen.

The lungs do not fill completely during inhalation or empty completely during exhalation. In normal, quiet breathing only approximately 10% of the air in the lungs is passed out to be replaced by the same amount of fresh air. This new air (tidal volume) mixes with the existing stale air (residual volume) already held in the lungs.

A man's lungs hold up to about 6 litres of air and a woman's about 4.25 litres. At rest about 400ml of air is taken into the lungs during normal inspiration. A deep breath can take in as much as 3-4 litres of air; during heavy exercise this can increase to almost 4.5 litres which is near the maximum of vital capacity. If a person is a shallow breather, carbon dioxide builds up in the body and this may be one of many causes of yawning.

The lung's volume can be influenced by different factors;

- larger volume is generally associated with taller people; people who live at higher altitude; fit people; younger people; and people who regularly sing or play woodwind/ brass instruments

- smaller volume is generally associated with shorter people; people who live at low altitude, obese people; and older people.

The Breathing Journey

Breathing in

Air/ oxygen breathed- in → throat → trachea/ windpipe →bronchial tubes → lungs → subdivision in lungs → bronchioles → air sac alveoli → alveoli capillary veins in their walls → blood → heart and then to rest of the body.

Breathing out

Carbon dioxide passes out from the blood through the alveoli and then the rest of journey is opposite to the breathing- in process.

Organs and structures affecting respiration

The structures, and their actions, of the different organs involved with respiration is simply described below. There are a number of excellent medical textbooks, health encyclopaedias and internet websites which can be consulted to gain further information of a much more detailed nature about their overall purposes and actions.

The Brain

The brain is the major organ of the nervous system. Together with the spinal cord it constitutes the central nervous system (CNS). The CNS controls basic functions such as breathing (respiration), heart rate and body temperature.

There are three main structures of the brain – the brainstem, cerebellum and the large forebrain (much of which is the cerebrum). The brainstem and cerebellum are the brain's oldest parts in evolutionary terms and it is the brainstem which is involved with the control of certain vital functions such as breathing and blood pressure. Breathing which is an automatic process is controlled by the respiratory centre contained in the brainstem's medulla.

The part of the brainstem which is significant for the automatic process of breathing is the medulla which contains the $9^{th} - 12^{th}$ cranial nerves and the vital centres which are groups of nerve cells involved in the automatic regulation of heart-beat, blood pressure and digestion as well as breathing.

Information about these functions are sent and received via the vagus nerve which is the 10th cranial nerve.

The vagus nerve is one of the most important components of the parasympathetic nervous system (which together with the sympathetic nervous system form the autonomic nervous system) which is concerned with maintaining the rhythmic automatic functioning of the internal body including the lungs.

It is the longest cranial nerve and amongst its branches which are concerned specifically with breathing are those to the larynx (voice box), pharynx (throat), trachea (wind-pipe) and lungs. Other of its branches are to the heart and main digestive organs.

The vagus nerve acts by releasing a chemical neurotransmitter Acetylcholine (Ach) which causes a narrowing of the bronchi and as it also supplies the larynx and trachea is involved in the actions of swallowing, coughing and sneezing.

While no conscious effort is needed to inhale or exhale air, the depth and rate of breathing can be altered voluntarily such as during exercise when internal organs and muscles make more demands for oxygen or when doing a meditative exercise or yoga session when there are less demands for oxygen.

Conscious breathing is controlled from the more evolved areas of the brain which are located in the cerebral cortex. When breathing is consciously controlled (such as when doing yoga or meditating) the cerebral cortex and the more evolved parts of the brain are stimulated.

Conscious breathing sends impulses from the cortex to the connecting areas that impact on emotions. Activating the cortex has a relaxing and balancing effect on the emotions. When breathing consciously, you are controlling which aspects of the brain dominate – causing consciousness to ascend from the primitive/ instinctive up to the evolved/ elevated.

The Nose, Mouth and the Paranasal Facial Sinuses

The **nose** is the uppermost part of the respiratory tract and is also the organ of smell. The nose has two nostrils at its front which are connected by a passage to the nasopharynx (which is the upper part of the throat) at its rear. This passage is divided into two chambers. Within the nose are three bony conchae projections which are each covered by mucous membrane.

The nose filters, warms and moistens inhaled air before it passes into the respiratory tract and is a protection against cold air because it has a warm humid interior. Just inside the nostrils, small hairs trap large dust particles and larger foreign bodies. Sneezing, which is a response to irritating substances, is induced to remove them. Smaller particles of dust are filtered from the inhaled air by the microscopic hairs on the surface of the conchae which is a narrow, curly shaped bone.

All air entering the nose passes over the blood vessels and mucus-secreting cells on the surface of the conchae. The mucus on the conchae flows inwards carrying harmful microorganisms and other foreign bodies back towards the nasopharynx so they can be ingested and destroyed by the stomach's gastric acid.

Air can also be inhaled and carbon dioxide gas exhaled through an open **mouth**. If air is inhaled through the mouth it will reach the pharynx airway but it won't have been filtered, warmed or moistened as it would have been if it had entered through the nose.

The nasal cavities, unlike the mouth, continuously produce the important molecule nitric oxide (NO) that increases blood flow through the lungs and also boost oxygen levels in the blood this is why it is important to breathe in through the nose rather than through an open mouth. The higher blood oxygen saturation can induce a feeling of being refreshed and provide greater endurance which can help people doing sports and other activities.

NO is produced in many parts of the body and as a signalling molecule it triggers different physiological effects. Its main respiratory benefits are the relaxation of smooth muscle in the airways (trachea and bronchioles) so making breathing easier and the promotion of blood flow to all organs. White blood cells and tissue macrophages produce NO for antimicrobial purposes which lead to the destruction of invading bacteria, viruses and parasites. Because NO is a gas it is often used as an inhaled therapy.

Because of its significance, the subject of NO is returned to in chapter five (page 7).

The bones which surround the nose are covered by air- filled mucous membrane lined cavities which are known as **paranasal sinuses**. The facial sinuses comprise the two frontal sinuses in the frontal bone of the forehead just above the eyebrows; the two maxillary sinuses in the cheekbones; two ethmoidal sinuses which are honeycomb-like cavities in bones between the nasal cavity and the eye sockets and the sphenoidal sinuses which are a collection of air spaces in the large winged bone behind the nose that forms the central part of the base of the skull. The sinuses lighten the skull, protect the brain and improve the voice's resonance.

Mucus drains from each sinus along a narrow channel that opens into the nose. It is a thick, slimy fluid secreted by mucous membranes. The purpose of the fluid is protective through keeping body structures moist and lubricated. It is produced and released on the membrane's surface by millions of specialised goblet cells which are situated within the membrane itself. Mucous is also found in the digestive, urinary and genital tracts.

Infection often spreads up, from the nose, via the sinus drainage channels and it may cause sinusitis which is an inflammation of the sinus lining. The maxillary sinuses in the cheekbones and the ethmoidal sinuses between the eyes are the most commonly affected. This condition usually results from a bacterial infection that develops as a complication of a viral infection such as the common cold. Other causes include upper tooth abscess, severe facial injury and forcing water up into the sinuses after jumping into cold water without covering the nose.

The symptoms of sinusitis include; a feeling of fullness in the affected area, a throbbing ache, stuffy nose, a stuffy nose, pain, formation of pus in the affected sinus(es) and a nasal discharge.

The airway between the nose and the trachea

Although the pharynx (or throat) is a relative short tube or airway between the back of the nose and the trachea it is complex in nature as there are a number of separate actions relating to respiration and digestion which are carried out by the structures within it. The pharynx is muscular and is lined with mucous membrane.

The first section of the pharynx is the passage (nasopharynx) connecting the nasal cavity behind the nose to the top of the throat behind the soft palate (whose purpose is to stop food ascending into the nose during swallowing).

The middle section of the pharynx is the oropharynx which is a passage for both food and air. It runs from the nasopharynx to below the tongue.

The lowest part of the pharynx is the laryngopharynx which is only a passage for food; it merges with the oesophagus.

The trachea

The trachea is the anatomical name for the windpipe and extends immediately down below from the larynx (the voice-box) for about ten centimetres to the point, behind the upper part of the sternum (breastbone), when it divides into two main bronchi which enter the two lungs.

The trachea is made up of fibrous & elastic tissue and smooth muscle. It also contains about twenty rings of cartilage which help keep the trachea open even during extreme neck movements.

In the chest, the trachea branches into two main bronchi which supply the left and right lungs.

The trachea's lining includes goblet cells which secrete mucus and other cells which bear minute, cell-like cilia which look like a coating of very small hairs. The mucus helps trap tiny particles in inhaled air such as dirt, germs, dust and other unwanted items that may otherwise end up in the lungs; the beating of the cilia moves the mucus and the particles upwards and out of the respiratory tract so helping keep the airway and lungs clear.

The lungs

The two lungs are the main organ of the body's respiration system. They supply the oxygen needed for the body's aerobic (requiring oxygen) metabolism and also eliminate the carbon dioxide waste product.

The two bronchi of the trachea enter the lungs (one in each) and subdivide into smaller bronchi and then into smaller bronchioles. The bronchial tubes are lined with billions of protective cilia, which resemble a coating of very small hairs, and by waving back and forth they spread mucus up into the throat from where it can be expelled out of the body. It is this (normally) protective mucus which cleans the lungs and rids them of dust, germs and other unwanted foreign bodies.

The bronchioles lead to air passages that open out into grape-like air sacs called alveoli (at birth there are approximately 20-50 million and in later life 300 - 480 million). It is through the many capillary veins in the thin walls of the alveoli that gases, notably oxygen during inspiration and carbon dioxide during expiration, respectively diffuse into or out of blood (The Gas Exchange as mentioned earlier).

An important action of the (cells of) alveoli is the secretion of a compound which is a surfactant. The surfactant has three functions and these are; the reduction of surface tension of pulmonary fluids, a contribution to the elastic properties of pulmonary tissue and the prevention of alveoli collapse especially when expiration happens.

The oxygen which enters the blood is carried to the heart and then pumped through the body to tissues and organs. While the oxygen is entering the bloodstream carbon dioxide waste gas passes from the blood through the alveoli and then out of the body.

The lungs are situated in the thoracic cavity in the chest behind the ribcage on either side of the heart. They are conically shaped at their apex and flatter at the base where they meet the diaphragm.

The right lung is shorter because the liver is below it and the left lung is narrower because of the vicinity of the heart.

The right lung has three lobes and the left lung has two lobes. These lobes are each made up of sponge-like tissue surrounded by a double membrane called the pleura (the pleural sack). This membrane allows the lungs to slide freely as they expand and contract during breathing and if one is punctured the other can continue working.

Lungs act like bellows and when they expand, they pull air (oxygen) into the body; when they compress, they expel waste carbon dioxide gas which is produced by the body. In the process of breathing, the air breathed-in contains 21% oxygen but the body only uses 5%; the rest is exhaled.

Lungs don't have their own muscles but rely on the diaphragm and rib cage to pump them.

At rest, a man's lungs can hold more air (750cc/ 1.5pints) than a woman's (285-393cc/ 0.6-0.8 pints). Healthy people without a chronic lung condition like bronchiectasis, even at maximum exercise intensity only use 70% of possible lung capacity.

Adults take about 15-20 breaths per minute which totals about 13 pints of air and about 20,000 breaths daily; an adult's average resting rate is 13-17 breaths per minute. A baby however, breathes at about 40 times/ minute. Children and women are usually faster breathers than men because their breathing rate is higher.

Lung capacity and lung function

Two important terms associated with the action of the lungs are lung function and lung capacity. Lung function is how the body uses oxygen contained in inhaled air and lung capacity is how much oxygen in inhaled air your body is able to use.

Lung capacity, which is the maximum amount of oxygen the body can use, can be improved with regular aerobic exercise (preferably three times weekly) and by other things such as better breathing, using flexibility exercises, giving up smoking, better posture and losing excess weight.

The lung's function cannot be recovered if it has been impaired. This function can be described as the ability of exchanging the two major gases (O_2 & CO_2) during breathing. It is determined by;

- how much air your lungs can hold
- how quickly you can take in and let air out from the lungs
- how well your lungs oxygenate to the blood supply and remove carbon dioxide from the blood supply.

There are a number of tests involved in the measurement of lung function and these include;

- the Pulmonary Function Test (PFT) which measures how well lungs work
- spirometry and lung volume tests which measure lung size and air flow
- tests which measure how well gases such as oxygen enter and exit blood
- pulse oximetry and arterial blood gas tests.

The diaphragm muscle and other muscles involved with breathing

This dome-shaped sheet of muscle separates the thorax (chest) from the abdomen which are two compartments with markedly different densities. It is attached to the spine, ribs and the sternum (breastbone). It is attached to the bottom of the rib cage. At rest, it extends upwards almost to nipple level.

In order for air to be drawn into the lungs during breathing - in (inhalation/ inspiration) the muscle fibres of the diaphragm contract so pulling the diaphragm downwards and making it flatten in shape. The intercostal muscles between the ribs contract and pull the rib-cage upwards and outwards. This movement increases the chest's volume, the lungs expand and air is sucked into them to fill the increased space. It is responsible for 70% of the work of inspiration. When it is contracted, the diaphragm presses down on the contents of the abdominal and outwards against the lower rib cage.

Other muscles associated with breathing-in include the pharyngeal muscles, the scalenes and sternomastoid in the neck; and shoulder, arm and trunk muscles especially when breathing becomes difficult.

When air is breathed- out (exhalation/expiration) the chest muscles and diaphragm relax, this causes the rib-cage to sink and the lungs to contract so squeezing out air.

The respiratory pump which ventilates the lungs, and so moves gas in and out of the lungs, is a collective term for the respiratory muscles, chest wall, nerves and respiratory centre.

The objectives of this chapter were;

1. **to give information about bronchiectasis and to outline details about its symptoms, diagnosis, treatments, prevention and research**
2. **to give a brief description of respiration, and the organs and structures which affect it.**

Suggested further reading

'Physiotherapy in Respiratory Care', Alexandra Hough; pub Springer-Science + Business Media BV, 2nd edition 1996; ISBN 9 781565 931312.

'Principles of Anatomy and Physiology', Tortora G.J. & Derrickson B; pub Wiley International; (15th edition), ISBN 978 1119400066.

CHAPTER 2: BEING POSITIVE

The Aims of this chapter are;

1. **to let the reader understand the importance of taking a positive approach towards the idea of using an alternative or supplementary self-treatment programme of their medical condition (in my case, bronchiectasis)**
2. **to consider how other outside agencies can help the individual on their path towards improved health**
3. **to see how different strategies can be adopted and used in the battle to achieve better health; how their results can be measured and why it is important to do this.**

Take charge of the situation

There are probably a number of bronchiectasis sufferers, who like me, don't see any perceptible improvement in their condition while taking antibiotics and/ or other medication and following physiotherapy advice and guidance. Many sufferers are also worried about the effects of taking repeated courses of antibiotics because of the well- publicised information that is being made available about the growing resistance to antibiotics by different bacteria and other pathogens.

Many people in either/ both of these groups are looking for different methods which could help them. These could either be additional to their existing treatment regime or have replaced parts of it.

By deciding to change their overall treatment approach, sufferers are stepping out of their comfort zone and are becoming more in charge of their (health) destiny. Sufferers/ patients if they adopt a new, individualistic & personal, positive approach to their own health care need to follow their new path for a reasonable length of time. This will allow them time to reflect on, and assess, their situation and will also deter them from becoming downhearted when there is no discernible short-term progress being made or when they hear hurtful comments from others who do not know about their situation.

If sufferers are undertaking changes to their existing treatment regime, they should discuss the proposed changes and their implications with their GP.

OK, so you have been troubled by a chest problem which you might have had for a long time since childhood into your 70s (or later) or you might have developed it later in life or have only had it as a young person for a short time. You have managed it reasonably well or it has got on top of you to an extent that you believe that it will overwhelm you no matter what you do to cope with, or combat, it especially by taking prescribed drug medication.

Your bronchiectasis symptoms probably aren't the same as everyone else's with this condition, but the incessant coughing up of sputum of different consistency or colour at different times is sure to figure high on your 'hit' list of intended improvements.

Your condition is likely to lead to frequent chest infections, tiredness and difficulties with concentration, breathlessness and possibly coughing up blood, sinus problems or incontinence leakage.

It's no wonder that these serious physical and emotional symptoms will lead many sufferers to develop stress, anxiety and even depression.

It is vital that a correct diagnosis, using the symptoms as the primary source, is made of any chest/ breathing condition is made as soon as possible. As well as confirming that it is bronchiectasis, it will rule out other possible conditions that the sufferer may be concerned about having such as bronchitis, COPD (chronic obstructive pulmonary disease), asthma or any other serious chest or breathing condition.

As soon as your condition has been diagnosed and confirmed as bronchiectasis, probably after seeing a specialist respiratory hospital consultant (or member of his/ her team), after referral by your GP following tests and scans at a hospital or clinic, you will learn what to do for the best for your health and wellbeing in the present and in the future.

The main aim for a sufferer of bronchiectasis should be to reduce the effects that the symptoms of the condition has on him/her and those around him/ her and to try to cope with this long- term condition with its changes, which include probable flare-ups.

Start by making a plan

Many sufferers will mentally decide to make a plan about how to proceed for the best and then physically flesh the plan out to include things such as aims, objectives and time scale. The plan however could simply be to follow what the 'doctor' says as he/ she is understandably understood as being the expert about the condition. As we have already seen the medical procedures, after the respiratory condition has been diagnosed, will usually mainly consist of prescribed antibiotics (especially during a 'flare-up' situation) or other medication often together with physiotherapy guidance including breathing exercises and how to clear the lungs of amassed sputum and advice on lifestyle changes.

It is important that any plan should include measurement tools, which could include a daily or weekly diary, to see if its aims have been achieved completely or in part. If all the aims have been achieved then very well done!! If only some of the aims have been achieved then again well done! In this latter case, or if few aims have been achieved, the plan can be revised and parts of it can be altered or discarded in favour of new methods and ideas.

When I decided to devise, and use, my own bronchiectasis self- treatment programme and methods I introduced a number of simple factors I could consider and measure to see if it had been successful. These were;

- the amount of phlegm/ sputum I coughed up during the day (and night)
- the colour and consistency of the phlegm I coughed up
- the approximate number and intensity of coughs I did during the day (and night)
- the number of tissues I used daily when coughing/ wiping away loosened phlegm
- the effects of my inhalation of asafoetida essential oil vapour and how the frequency of doing this is influenced by the condition of the lungs
- my daily SATS oxygen saturation level reading. Oxygen saturation is a measure of how much of the haemoglobin in the blood is carrying oxygen. Normal rate of SPO2 levels are 90-100%; ideally it should be above 95%. I take my reading, at the beginning of the day before getting out of bed, using a small SATS/ pulse oximeter which is attached to the first finger of the left hand (the resting pulse can be recorded at the same time)
- my ability to do physical activities such as regular gymnasium workouts, gardening and daily dog walking and the varying amounts of energy that has to be expended on different days. Other sufferers will obviously carry out different types and levels of physical activities and exercise to me depending on their health condition, age, gender etc
- my concentration levels, degree of tiredness and sleep pattern
- my physical and mental health and how I felt at any time.

Give thanks to others

If by using medical intervention (e.g. taking prescribed antibiotics) and by following physiotherapists' guidance the symptoms of the bronchiectasis are kept under control then the situation is seen as being stable. At this time, thanks should be given that the drugs are available and that medical knowledge and personnel were available to facilitate the stabilisation of the situation. By appreciating the medical help being given, the sufferer will automatically feel more positive about things and negativity will be reduced in his/her mind.

Positivity is contagious and it should be helpful to sufferers for it to reinforced by input from those around them – family, friends and work colleagues. These people will think and act in an uplifting way and their energy should lift the sufferer's spirits. It could be valuable to show them any diary that you might keep which shows how you have progressed and the work that you have done to try to improve health wise.

Because others' help can be vital, it is a great idea that they be thanked and one way to do this is to celebrate with them your successes. Both you and they will mutually benefit from this as it will show why their help is so necessary and valued.

Positive thinking techniques

People can either think positively ('a glass half full') or negatively ('a glass half empty') about any problem they are having to face or overcome. Obviously, at times it is necessary for a neutral 'grounded' approach to be adopted.

If thoughts are positive and uplifting then it is more possible that many health conditions such as bronchiectasis can be coped with better. The opposite may occur if negative ideas or thoughts get the upper hand.

As the state of someone's health should be thought of as the most important thing in their life, positive thoughts about ways of improved coping with bronchiectasis, which is a major part of their overall health problems, should be in their mind throughout the waking hours.

Often people only think about and value their good health when something goes wrong e.g. breaking a leg while playing football or falling off a ladder. If this traumatic event happens the unfortunate person has to 'fire fight' to try to make their situation better.

By adopting a positive attitude and with an improvement in self-confidence, most people will improve their mood and outlook and this will help them stay motivated to stay on the path of improvements such as increasing lung capacity.

As well as only filling the mind with positive thoughts, a sufferer could also just use positive words and phrases in conversation. Negative words should be forgotten as much as possible. It doesn't hurt to be a 'smiley' person even on days when smiling at life is hard to do. Others looking at your smiles will usually adopt a happy, positive view of you and be more willing to try to help you.

Meditation

Often negative thoughts and thinking will happen in cycles. Something can happen and it will depress you to an extent that everything becomes tainted with a negative brush. Daily meditation can be a tool to break the cycle and allow the mind to become refocused.

It allows the mind to clear and we can think logically about life without being distracted by everything happening around you. If negative thinking is taking over the mind then this is the time to stop and meditate even if it is for a few minutes. The calmness meditation brings, will allow someone get back to reality, and thought processes can again become balanced.

Meditation can be accessed through the internet but it is probably better to find a good teacher who will lead guided meditations in either a group setting or on an individual basis. A good introduction to meditation (and yoga) is in a holiday setting at a health spa or at a retreat. Personal recommendations and previous participants' internet comments about teachers and meditation classes / holidays can be very helpful to anyone wanting to learn meditation. There are also a number of UK meditation associations whose contact details can be found on the internet.

Better overall health and improved lifestyle

Although this book's chapter concentrates on the relationship between mental positivity and the fight-back against bronchiectasis, and its symptoms, there is no doubt that overall health and wellbeing, including the reduction of stress, of sufferers can be helped by realising the importance of a healthy diet, sensible drinking, appropriate exercising and sound sleeping and acting on these aspects of a good lifestyle.

If someone takes steps to adopt or improve their existing lifestyle, this should include a mental discipline menu of no/ low intake of alcohol, no recreational drugs or substances and no smoking; this will be a great positive step in someone taking control of his/ her health.

If overall health can be improved, this will allow a sufferer to specifically allocate more effort in time and money on combatting bronchiectasis and its effects.

Breathing clubs and slimming clubs

There are many national charities with local groups and the NHS which can help people with respiratory conditions. Additionally, voluntary breathing clubs have been set up which offer education and exercise opportunities to its members. Suitable participants for these clubs are usually referred by interested GPs and if this help (which is usually free or at low cost) is available then take advantage of it. A good example in the Shrewsbury, Shropshire area is a breathing group which before the COVID-19 outbreak met socially with participants having a short talk, use of a supervised gym and playing badminton and table tennis together – a wonderful example.

If people's respiratory problems are caused, or exacerbated, by obesity there are schemes whereby a GP may refer their suitable patients to a local slimming club for advice and support in losing weight sensibly.

Increased sociability is an important part of the value of joining and regularly using breathing clubs and slimming clubs.

Information providers and sources

The public library can be a good resource for getting information and books about how to eat healthily on a low (or high) income. Libraries, on their community notice board, often publicise courses and meetings which help people improve their health, general lifestyle and cooking skills.

The internet and health & spiritual based magazines are other reference sources for people to learn about positivity and also how to improve their physical, mental and emotional health.

Social Prescribing

Some GPS and their practice nurse are now able to refer suitable patients for Social Prescribing. This is a non-medical programme where the patients work with a trained advisor who helps people understand their health and wellbeing needs and supports them in setting realistic goals and developing and following up an action plan which will achieve these.

Many people taking part in this programme are;

- living with a long-term (chronic) health condition like bronchiectasis
- wanting to change their lifestyle e.g. giving up smoking or losing weight
- feeling worried, anxious or depressed
- feeling lonely, socially isolated or embarrassed by their health condition.

Good sleep

The importance of good sleep in combatting stress and its associated problems has long been accepted. A good bed and bedding including correct pillows are a must, with the mattress being changed at least about every eight years. I use only one very flat pillow when I sleep as I feel that this keeps my neck in a neutral position. If the bed's head and feet ends can be electrically adjusted this will assist the technique of postural drainage which has been designed to help clear excess sputum from the airways.

Other things to help encourage good sleep include;

- ✓ the introduction of fresh air ventilation by leaving a window slightly ajar
- ✓ using 'blackout' curtains to reduce light in the bedroom from outside
- ✓ no intake of caffeine in a few hours before going to bed
- ✓ no use of 'screens' on the television, radio, computer/laptop, mobile cell phones or other 'tech' equipment in the bedroom in the hour before 'lights out'
- ✓ wearing comfortable sleepwear clothing made of natural fibres.

Physical activity and exercise

Perhaps an important tool in helping to retain a positive approach to thinking is to undertake physical activity consistently and regularly. During exercise the brain produces chemicals called endorphins which give the mind and body a natural 'high' (long distance runners have often said that they have experienced this emotional and physical feeling).

There is also a psychological boost from setting an exercise goal and following it through – this could range from completing a charity long - distance bike ride fund raising event or simply getting your garden back into shape after it has been neglected for a long time. Feeling better and happier after exercising can also boost confidence and mood.

Whilst doing physical exercise the mind is distracted from worrying about troubling matters which are often the causes of fear, anxiety and depression.

The benefits of taking exercise or doing activities to help reduce the effects of stress and some mental conditions is now being recognised more widely. One example is the recent initiative between the Royal Horticultural Society and the NHS to examine the physical, mental and emotional health values of gardening. Some GPs now view gardening as a treatment option.

Many GP practices also support various exercise activities for those with physical, mental and emotional health problems These activities including gentle walking groups and walking football and walking netball sessions. Details of these can be found at the GP practice.

For those people who are not interested in sport or walking there are many groups such as local 'knit and natter' knitting groups and choirs which offer social interaction. Singing and acting groups bring the practical benefits of improved breathing through their performances and rehearsals.

It is important to gradually increase controlled exercise tolerance whatever type of exercise or activity is being undertaken. Exercise causes heart and breathing rates to increase. This will lead to the heart and lungs being strengthened with additional oxygen being pumped around the body via the blood circulation system. It is possible to achieve a lung capacity increase of 5 – 15% with a regular cardio exercise programme.

A good example of the benefit of exercise is by completing a specialised supervised hospital pulmonary rehabilitation (PR) programme and continuing with this type of exercise afterwards. As well as addressing breathlessness problems, this type of tailored exercise programme will help many sufferers come out of a cycle of inactivity which can lead to fear, anxiety and depression.

The Depression/ Inactivity Circle

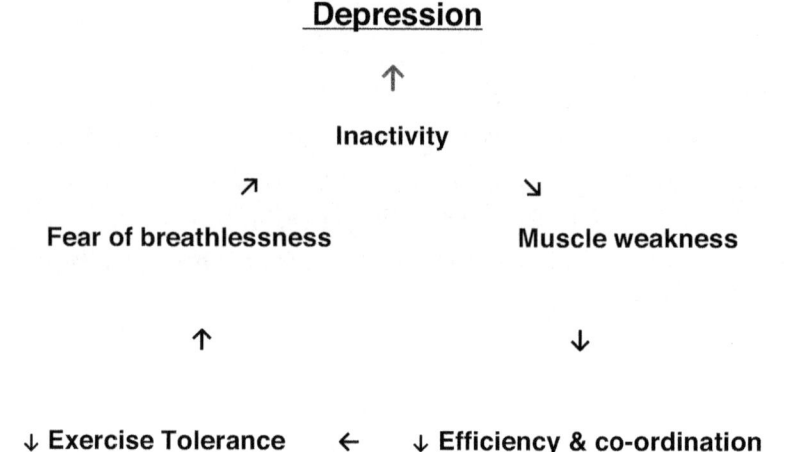

Depression

↑

Inactivity

↗ ↘

Fear of breathlessness   **Muscle weakness**

↑ ↓

↓ **Exercise Tolerance** ← ↓ **Efficiency & co-ordination**

Costs, and Equipment needed, for activities and exercise

Costs of carrying out physical activity and exercise vary from none (taking a walk around your garden, public park or accessible countryside) through to expensive (joining exclusive country or health clubs or sports clubs). It is important that correct footwear and clothing are worn when undertaking any form of physical activity and that outdoors in very cold weather a mouth covering such as a scarf should be worn and deep breathing be avoided to prevent cold air reaching the lungs.

Improving breathing

As breathing is improved by increasing its efficiency, this will have a beneficial effect on the body's overall functioning by increasing the supply of oxygen to all its organs and structures via the blood supply.

Breathing can be improved by taking regular exercise and by doing strenuous (if possible) physical activity. It is thought that lung capacity which is the maximum amount of oxygen (O_2) the body can use, can be improved by 5-15% with regular aerobic (with oxygen) exercise workouts or serious swimming sessions. Self- confidence will help to encourage someone to keep to any health or regular exercise plan and the advantage of doing exercise with a friend or 'buddy' is often mentioned.

Specific and targeted breathing exercises can help and as well as those taught by specialised respiratory physiotherapists there are a number of techniques which can be self- taught; from books, by viewing tuition sites on the internet or by working with a qualified fitness/ personal trainer in a gym, at home or in a work location.

Breathing should be improved by;

- ✓ living, working and doing leisure activities in environments which should be as clean as possible
- ✓ avoid applying, or breathing-in, strongly smelling perfume and body products

- ✓ the home being cleaned to remove dust pollutants and dust mites and harmful cleaning products should be avoided
- ✓ at work, safety clothing and masks with replacement filters should be worn when needed, especially when dangerous materials such as asbestos is being removed
- ✓ when gardening, wear a mask if pruning large trees, shrubs and climbers (such as ivy) and consider wetting their dusty surfaces before starting work.
- ✓ if it is really necessary, only spray plants on a still day – this advice should also apply to agricultural operations.

More information about improving breathing and breathing methods in given in chapter 5.

Diet and Posture

Improved posture will bring many positive health advantages including the reduction of stress on the lungs. Any planned weight loss will also help available oxygen to be used more efficiently and will help general health.

Bronchiectasis as well as other conditions such as asthma, cancer, diabetes and arthritis are associated with a low vitamin D level. Intake can be boosted by good sunlight exposure and by having a balanced diet including; oily fish such as salmon, sardines and tuna; red and white meat; liver; egg yolks and fortified foods such as some fat spreads and breakfast cereals. Vitamin D supplements can be used, including by vegetarians and vegans.

Smoking and Vaping

Finally, last but certainly not least, it is imperative to stop smoking and also not start doing it. There are a number of available products like nicotine patches which can help a smoker reduce and then give up the habit. The recent introduction and 'vaping' use of E-cigarettes has been seen as a weapon against smoking (although their clouds of smoke are very anti-social to others nearby). The health risks of vaping are still being evaluated and certain countries and states in the USA have limited or banned their use. There is a lot of help available through the GP surgery which can also help a smoker give up. This advice about smoking also applies to people who smoke recreational drugs like cannabis.

Please remember that it is not only the smoker's overall health, including the lungs and respiration, which can be damaged by smoking but also the health of those around him/her who are affected by the passive smoking of tobacco smoke. This is especially relevant to those whose lungs are really vulnerable such as the foetus, baby, toddler and young people and who are unable to take decisions and look after themselves.

Persevere with changes to the old regime

It is important to keep to any new regime and not be put off if planned improvements do not occur as quickly as you hoped. There is no easy path to success and the improvements to my own bronchiectasis and its symptoms have taken about two years to accomplish and during that time I have had my ups and downs; successes and setbacks. Mine has been a long haul indeed with more work ongoing but my struggle, which has resulted in a 'very bright light at the end of my recovery tunnel', has been <u>very</u> worthwhile.

It is important to realise as I did that there will be many obstacles to progress but that these can usually be overcome.

Know when to revert back to the old regime

If someone follows my self-help programme and the methods I have developed they can always remember that they can at any time take a step back and return back to their original medical treatment regime if the feel no benefit is being gained.

There is no shame in reverting - you will have the knowledge that for at least a while you have tried to take more responsibility for your health care and have tried simply not to rely on unending courses of antibiotics and other drugs, with the uncomfortable side effects they often bring, and respiratory physiotherapy techniques.

POSITIVITY ACTION PLAN

1. **TAKE CHARGE OF THE SITUATION**
2. **MAKE A PLAN**
3. **GIVE THANKS TO OTHERS**
4. **USE POSITIVE THINKING TECHNIQUES**
5. **DEVELOP BETTER OVERALL HEALTH & IMPROVED LIFESTYLE**
6. **UNDERSTAND THE IMPORTANCE OF PHYSICAL ACTIVITY**
7. **IMPROVE YOUR BREATHING**
8. **PERSEVERE WITH CHANGES TO THE OLD REGIME**
9. **BUT HOWEVER, KNOW WHEN TO REVERT BACK TO THE OLD REGIME.**

The Objectives of this chapter were;

1. **to realise that positivity is a necessary step in trying to come to terms with bronchiectasis and that a self-help treatment regime is a possible way to improve the situation**
2. **to learn that organisations and close family/ colleagues/ friends are important as part of a team support effort to help strengthen an individual's resolve and commitment. Thanks, should be directed back to others where necessary**
3. **to show that improvements to overall health, as well as to any specific health condition such as**

bronchiectasis, are essential for positive physical, mental and emotional development
4. to understand the great importance of physical activity and better breathing to improving health conditions. The social side of exercising and activities and their beneficial effects should not be underestimated
5. to realise that if any new self-help treatment regime is not successful there is no shame associated with reverting back to the previous conventional form of treatment if it is a better option.

CHAPTER 3: USING ASAFOETIDA ESSENTIAL OIL

The Aims of this chapter are;

1. to describe how I use (ferula) asafoetida essential oil vapour in an easy to do self-treatment session(s) to help me cope with, and improve the condition of, my bronchiectasis.
2. to inform the reader about the generally little-known asafoetida plant, and its many benefits. This plant has been used for thousands of years for many widespread medical problems & conditions; in cuisines and in horticulture and agriculture.

Introduction

Using (ferula) asafoetida essential oil vapour

I described in the introduction that it was by chance that I read in a good friend's copy of an encyclopaedia of aromatherapy oils by Julia Lawless about the existence of the plant called asafoetida -its properties, healing actions, production and history.

I was extremely lucky to have seen a reference to this herbal plant as it is rarely mentioned in a great many aromatherapy text books unlike more common, better known aromatherapy plant sources such as eucalyptus, lavender pine, thyme, fennel, myrrh, ginger and hyssop etc which are more regularly used for respiratory conditions (and many other conditions) by qualified aromatherapists and others.

My interest in, and importance to me of, asafoetida is that this plant is reputed to treat various respiratory ailments including bronchiectasis, bronchitis, asthma and whooping cough in addition to many other conditions including stress & nervous tension, constipation and flatulence.

Although there are a great number of other essential oils which have been used for hundreds, if not thousands, of years to help conditions of the respiratory system I was drawn to the use of asafoetida to see if it would help my bronchiectasis and its symptoms.

Having discovered an unusual herb which could possibly help me treat my bronchiectasis I had to decide how to use it safely. The alternative options were;

- some drops of the asafoetida essential oil added to a bath
- some drops of the oil to be used during an aromatherapy massage
- some drops of the oil vaporised in a room in a burner or diffuser or in a bowl of water placed on a warm radiator
- some drops of the oil to be inhaled as a vapour after being added to hot (not boiling) water.

Because asafoetida has a very strong, unpleasant odour with a bitter acrid taste it certainly fulfils one of its synonym descriptions as 'Devil's Dung'. I therefore decided that I would choose the final option as the other three alternatives are very antisocial.

Accordingly, I decided to do the inhalations, in a well ventilated space in my outside garage (well away from my wife) as it was better for its aroma, which lingers for a long time, to be better kept outside the house rather than indoors!

Nose, throat and lung infections are conditions which can often respond very well to treatments with the vapour of essential oils. Not only are the properties of the oil directed to the lungs but they cause increased bronchial secretion which is a protective reaction.

Inhalation gives the fastest absorption into the respiratory system through being introduced into the lungs. It is the action of components such as the disulphides in this volatile oil which aid the coughing up of congested mucus.

My asafoetida oil inhalation session

Asafoetida essential oil can be purchased from a reputable supplier -either directly at some herbariums or health stores or through an established supplier through the internet. It is recommended that companies used are members of a recognised trade organisation; in the UK; these are the British Essential Oil Association (www.beoa.co.uk) and the British Herb Trade Organisation (www.bhta.org.uk)

The bottle containing the oil should be stored in a dark place, with its lid tightly shut, away from the reach of young children or pets. It is probably financially prudent in the first instance to purchase the smallest amount available as this will enable the buyer to get used to carrying out inhalations and to see whether they are producing positive results. If inhalations are going well, a larger volume bottle can be purchased thereafter as this will probably be more cost effective and financially beneficial.

In a container, such as a small bowl, add a few drops of the essential oil to hot water ensuring that none is spilt on the skin or in the eyes (if this happens bathe the affected area or eyes with cold water). The mixture is then inhaled through the nose with the mouth shut at a distance of about 18 inches above the container with the liquid mixture. Exhalation is done through an open mouth. Because the oil's odour is retained by the container it is advisable to keep using only this receptacle.

If a child is doing an inhalation this should be done under the close supervision of an adult.

It is likely that after a short time, some phlegm will be loosened in the airways and if this happens it must be coughed out into a handy, nearby disposable tissue. Very often, sinus and nasal congestion will also be addressed and reduced. Both during and after the session the need to blow the nose is very likely to be stimulated – have plenty of tissues available to cope with this eventuality.

It is not necessary to cover the head with a cloth during any inhalation session, which is often the recommended case with inhalations. A cloth would retain the smell of the asafoetida and the vapour will work well anyway without a cloth covering the head.

After a short time, probably five or six minutes, the amount, colour and consistency of the phlegm should change and diminish. At this point it is probably best to stop the session as this will reduce the risk of chest soreness.

At the end of the session, the used tissues should be disposed of hygienically.

When the mixed oil & water solution has cooled it can be used in a spray as a natural pesticide on garden plant insect pests such as blackfly or cherry beetles. A friend and I have independently used some and have found it to be very effective.

If not being used as a natural pesticide, the cooled mixture can be disposed of by possibly either being carefully thrown on to a flower bed or poured into a closable waste container. It should not be poured down a drain and because the mixture contains oil it will mark stonework if it is spilt on it – however this can be removed with speedy, correct cleaning. If the essential oil is spilt on clothing this should be washed separately from other items and not in a washing machine because of its lingering noxious odour.

During the inhalation session, a music source such as radio or CD player can play background music. This will have the dual functions of firstly, masking any noise made by any stimulated coughing or clearing of the throat and nose while doing the inhalation. Secondly, this could be a basic way of timing a session i.e. if the same results are achieved when two records are played on the radio as when three records are played this will indicate that an improvement in the respiratory system is being achieved. Obviously, a watch or clock can be used for timing.

When the inhalation sessions start, they can be done once, twice or three times daily if time permits and no chest soreness is caused by them. After a few days of repeated inhalations, it is likely that the need to do them will diminish and it could be that there becomes a longer time interval between inhalations. This will be different for each individual; I have now gone to a break of four - six weeks before having another inhalation.

It is useful to keep a diary or record about the inhalations to include their duration; the need to cough; the amount of coughing and the production of phlegm/mucus (and its colour & consistency) during the inhalation; and how the symptoms of the bronchiectasis are affected by the inhalation. By doing this, a sufferer can be given confidence to continue the inhalations if improvements are being noted or stop doing them if they don't improve things.

When I commenced doing the inhalations I did them for the first week up to three times daily and the frequency gradually reduced. My body had 'told' me that this dramatic reduction was appropriate because the marked improvement in my condition was such that I had not needed to clear my lungs or cough as much. I rely on my body to 'tell' me when I need an inhalation and its message is usually right.

It is important to work to a routine and give it a reasonable time to work as I did; try not to skip the necessary (possibly daily at the beginning) inhalation(s) unless there is a good reason to do so.

When not to use asafoetida oil vapour

My own experience

When reading books about any medical treatment or therapy – conventional or complementary, there will always be a mention of contraindications to its usage which is designed to both protect and inform the 'patient' and the practitioner. Following convention this book is no different, and caution about when to use asafoetida essential oil should be considered.

I am pleased to say that I have not experienced any harmful health side effects from inhaling asafoetida oil vapours on many occasions over several years.

Additionally, I must say on this important subject, that in the past seven months (at the time of writing) I have had two successful hip replacement operations at the internationally renowned Robert Jones & Agnes Hunt orthopaedic hospital in Oswestry. My inhalation of the asafoetida essential oil vapour was closely questioned by their pharmacy and I agreed to stop using it for a couple of weeks before each operation was due to take place. However due to unforeseen circumstances, my first operation was rescheduled and brought forward and, in the event, I was only able to stop using the oil 36 hours before the operation. On the day my SATS oxygen haemoglobin level was 99%; my anaesthetist was happy with my condition and this operation proceeded without a hitch and was successful.

Before the second operation, which again was rescheduled, I stopped using the oil only one day before the operation. Again, the anaesthetist was satisfied with my breathing condition and SATS levels both before and during the operation (which was again successful).

Conventional safety contraindications

When considering some of the contraindications listed below, potential users may also be interested in and influenced by some of the information given later in this chapter, together with my experience described above, before deciding whether they should inhale the oil vapour to address their own bronchiectasis). Conventionally it is not recommended for;

- ❖ women in the first trimester of their pregnancy or for those trying to get pregnant (this advice also applies to most essential oils). Similarly, breast feeding mothers shouldn't use asafoetida as its constituent chemicals may pass on to the infants
- ❖ children under five years of age
- ❖ people who are suffering from any type of bleeding disorder
- ❖ persons of an Ayurvedic 'Pitta' type temperament

- ❖ alcoholics
- ❖ people suffering from hyperacidity and gastric ulcers
- ❖ people suffering nerve related disorders who may be predisposed to having seizures
- ❖ people who are to undergo serious elective surgery, such as a major joint replacement, will be advised during their pre-operative assessment to cease using this (or any other) essential oil about two weeks before the operation because it could either affect the efficacy of the anaesthetic or the blood clotting process. This advice is given to many patients who use any form of complementary medicine because testing of complementary medicines is of a different standard to that afforded to conventional medicines. If this is the situation, it could be that the patient could transfer back to an approved, tested medical drug for the short period before the operation and then return to their complementary medicine at a safe period after the operation (this subject can be discussed with the surgeon or anaesthetist prior to the surgery).

If any adverse health conditions arise from using the oil then you should stop using it immediately.

What is asafoetida?

The species asafoetida belongs to the celery family Apiaceae (Umbelliferae) and is correctly titled Ferula assa-foetida, it also has a number of synonyms (other names) and spellings by which it is known and which can be confusing to members of the public.

It is a large, branching, herbaceous perennial, monoecious (having unisexual organs or flowers on a single plant/ herb) and is one of the most important of the 130 species of Ferula; only some of these species yield the asafoetida *(Santapau & Henri 1973, Scitech Journal ISSN 2347 -7318)*. Currently there are only about eight known species of ferula which are traded in the middle and near east as a source of asafoetida and other oleo-gum resin.

It grows up to 3m (9.75 feet) high with a circular mass of 30-40cms (12-16 ins) leaves. Flowering stems are 2.5-3m high and 10cms (3.9 ins) thick and hollow. They contain a number of ducts in the cortex which contain the (active) resinous gum. It is not harvested until it is at least four years old.

Its flowers are pale greenish yellow and fruits are oval, flat, thin and reddish brown which produce a milky juice with a strong smell. Roots and rhizomes are thick, massive and pulpy and are the main source of the plant's oleo- gum resin, this gum is similar to that contained in the stems.

All parts of the plant have a distinctive fetid smell.

The English name (Ferula) asafoetida is derived from the Latin 'ferula' which means carrier or vehicle; 'asa' which is a Latinised form of the Persian Farsi 'aza' means mastic resin; and the Latin word 'foetidus' means smelling/ fetid which refers to the herb's strong sulphurous smell. Asafoetida is also alternatively known as asafetida in English.

In Iran, the country with the highest production, asafoetida is translated as Angustha- Gandha.

As mentioned previously, it has a number of synonym names including; gum asafedita, devil's dung (a name originally given by Germans), 'stinking gum', 'devil's sweat' (Turkish), 'merde du Diable' (French), A-wei (Chinese), hing and giant fennel. A common translation of the Hindi word Hing which is also known as Hingu and Heeng in parts of India is 'Food of the Gods'.

The other main species from which asafoetida is extracted is *F.narthex* Boiss which is much smaller (1.5 – 2 m high) with smaller leaves and fruit.

As well as having medicinal properties, asafoetida is now more commonly used as a spice in cooking in many different cuisines throughout the world.

Where is asafoetida grown?

The perennial asafoetida plant is native to the region between the Mediterranean and Central Asia. Especially in eastern Iran (including the regions of Khorasan, Baluchistan and Kerman), Uzbekistan, the Kyrgyz republic, Western Afghanistan, Turkey, Russia and in the Zagros and Alburz mountain chain up to the Persian Gulf. Its habitats are mainly desert and mountains at an altitude of 190-2,400 m on slopes of 15-70% with an annual precipitation of 250-350mm (*Shad 1995, quoted Nadjafi et al., 2006*).

A few other ferula species which produce asafoetida are cultivated in other regions of south-west Asia such as Pakistan, Tibet, Kashmir; and Jammu and some parts of the Punjab in India. In Afghanistan it grows between 600 – 1200 m above sea level.

The species of ferula which produce the oleo-resin have been listed by *Dutt (1928), Coppen (2005) and Farooqui (2008).*

There are two main varieties of asafoetida – Hing Kabuli Sufaid (milky white asafoetida) and Hing Lal (red/ black asafoetida).

White asafoetida has a strong smell, and a crystalline form which gives it the description 'diamond like' asafoetida. This type has a more medicinal value. The blackish type is used in cooking and adds an unusual and delicate flavour to dishes.

India is the major consumer of asafoetida in its culinary spice form. About 70% of the world's production is consumed there for both culinary and medicinal purposes (some of which is re-exported). Historically India has imported asafoetida from Iran, Turkey, Kashmir, Western Tibet and Pakistan's, Baltistan and Astore regions.

At the time of writing (August 2020) it is difficult to obtain supplies of asafoetida from Iran. A current alternative source for the UK essential oil industry is from Uzbekistan.

How is asafoetida produced?

Asafoetida is extracted as a dried latex (gum oleoresin) which is derived from a milky sap which is produced by making repeated incisions into the plant's 4 – 5 years old thick and pulpy rhizome or tap root just above ground level in March and April, before the start of its flowering season. This carrot-shaped root is laid bare and the stem cut off close to the crown.

This incision process is repeated several times for up to three months, at intervals of about 10 days, until exudation/leakage stops. Between each incision, the exposed root is covered by a dome-shaped structure made from twigs, stones and earth; this covering is then scraped off and a fresh slice is cut to produce more latex. There may be a yield of 2lbs or more of gum resin. Research by *Khosrogerdi (1999)* has shown that four incisions, over a three months period, is the best harvesting method for plant productivity and growth.

The fresh resinous, milky, sappy juice when it leaks out is greyish-white but with age darkens and hardens into dark amber reddish, then yellow and finally brown lumps on contact with the air. These lumps are then scraped off and collected. Because this resin is difficult to grate it is traditionally crushed between stones or with a hammer.

Harvesting methods of the oleo- gum resin varies between countries.

Dried sap which is extracted from the black type of asafoetida's stem and root is used as the culinary spice.

Before being sold, the oleoresin is often mixed up with a larger volume of red clay or similar substitutes such as gum Arabic, wheat flower, rice flour or turmeric. The most commonly available type is compounded asafoetida which is a fine powder containing 30% resin mixed together with any of gypsum, red clay, chalk, barley rice flour, potato flour, white wheat flour, or/and gum arabic.

Asafoetida is available in three forms i.e. 'Tears', 'Mass' and 'Paste'. 'Tears' is the purest form of resin which is flattened or rounded, 5-30mm in diameter and a greyish or dull yellow in colour, it can retain its original colour for several years. It is the 'Tears' form that is sold in Chinese pharmacies (it may have fragments of root and surrounding earth).

'Mass' asafoetida is the most common available in the market and is a mass of 'Tears' mixed with fragments of soil. 'Paste' also contains soil and woody material.

Some ferula species such as *F. galbaniflua Boiss* and F. *Buhse (*named after F.A. Buhse a German traveller in the 1840s) produce Galbanum which is mixed with the asafoetida, and these are used to a limited extent as perfume fixatives. Its essential oil is then obtained from the resin by the steam distillation method. An absolute, resinoid and tincture are also produced. The oil is yellow- orange which has a bitter and acrid taste with a strong odour similar to garlic. However, beneath the odour there is a sweet, balsamic note.

Asafoetida is stored in sealed plastic containers because its odour is so strong that it could contaminate other foods stored nearby if the container is not airtight.

Actions of asafoetida

Asafoetida has a number of actions and it is;

- ✓ antispasmodic (relieves or cures spasms of smooth muscles)
- ✓ carminative (relieves flatulence and gripping pain in the stomach and intestines)
- ✓ expectorant (promotes the secretion of sputum through the air passages e.g. used to treat coughs)
- ✓ hypotensive (reduces blood pressure)
- ✓ stimulating (increases physiological activity).

Other actions include it being; anti-inflammatory, diuretic, antibacterial, aphrodisiac, analgesic, antiviral, laxative, diuretic, aphrodisiac, emmenagogue (stimulates or increases menstrual flow) and nerve stimulating.

Its odour repels most animals (and people as well!). However, looking at a number of UK websites, asafoetida in both essential oil or flakes/powder form is a very attractive lure for carp when mixed with other bait components by carp fishermen.

Principal constituents of asafoetida

Like most plants, and their essential oils, asafoetida is extremely complex in its composition.

As well as treating respiratory conditions it is thought that asafoetida could be helpful for;

- ✓ treating insect bites (when mixed as a paste)
- ✓ headache relief by improving blood flow which can help tension and pain
- ✓ toothache and earache treatment because of its anti-inflammatory, analgesic and antibacterial effects
- ✓ lowering blood pressure
- ✓ improving digestive problems
- ✓ analgesia
- ✓ boosting fertility
- ✓ improving reproductive health
- ✓ nervous disorders such as mood swings, chronic anxiety, depression and stress.

Information about, and measurements of, asafoetida vary but the most commonly quoted are those contained in the paper *'Ferula asafoetida: Traditional uses and pharmacological activity'*, Mahendra P and Bisht S, Pharmacogn Rev. 2012 Jul-Dec; 6 (12() 141-146.

They found that;

1. per 100 gms of asafoetida it consisted of;
   - carbohydrates 67.8%
   - moisture 16%
   - minerals and vitamins 7%
   - protein 4%
   - dietary fibre 4.1%
   - fat 1.1%
2. minerals – substantial calcium, phosphorus & iron
3. vitamins – carotene, riboflavin & niacin
4. a calorific value of 297 which contains;
   - 40-64% resinous material – ferulic acid, umbelliferone, asaresinotannols, farnesiferols A, B & C
   - 25% gum – glucose, galactose, l-arabinose, rhamnose & glucuronic acid
   - 3 – 17% volatile oils – disulphides as its major components (notably, 2-butyl propenyl disulphide (E & Z - isomers), monoterpenes (α and β- pinene, etc), free ferulic acid, valeric acid and traces of vanillin minerals 7% 40-64% resin; 25% endogeneous gum; 10-17% volatile oil; and 1.5 -10% ash.
5. Bioactive (having a biological effect on living tissue) components of the oleoresin and gum (25% of plant weight) include;

- Ferulsinaic acid
- Ferulic acid (the main phyto-chemical which is 40-60% of the gum has a number of properties including being anti-cancerous, hepato (liver)-protective, antioxidant and anti-inflammatory)
- 2-Butyl propenyl disulphide & Diallyl disulphide – these are odorous compounds
- Umbelliferone
- Foetidin
- Luteolin
- Phenolic compound
- Kamolonol
- Valeric.

In Mahendra & Bisht's paper, a valuable table is included which shows a comprehensive list of over 30 different pharmacological activities (e.g. antiviral, anticancer, anti -HIV etc) of the different chemical constituents found in the asafoetida gum resin. The effects of different clinical trials and the pharmacological activities of ferula asafoetida in the following fields were listed;

➢ the gastro intestinal tract
➢ cancer
➢ women's ailments and conditions
➢ gene expression
➢ effect on blood pressure and relaxation
➢ hypersensitivity
➢ lipid profile
➢ hepatoprotective (liver) effect
➢ CNS (central nervous system) and the heart
➢ blood sugar level regulation.

Amongst the conclusions of this paper, it was acknowledged that traditionally all over the world ferula asafoetida has been used for the treatment of a number of diseases and conditions. Recent pharmacological and biological studies have shown that asafoetida possesses a number of qualities which can be utilised for the treatment of many significant conditions including cancer, diabetes and raised arterial blood pressure.

Asafoetida seemingly therefore has great medical significance and like the authors of many other papers there is a need for more detailed studies of asafoetida in complex clinical trials.

As well as the paper by *Mahendra and Bisht* there have been a significant number of other investigative papers and reports into the constituents of asafoetida.

Possibly the most significant of these was that of *Kavoosi G and Rowshan V* in their paper *'Chemical composition, antioxidant and antimicrobial activities of essential oil obtained from Ferula assa-foetida oleo-gum-resin; effect of collection time' pub. Food Chem, Vol 138, issue 4, 15.6. 2013, pages 2180 -2187*. They found that additional constituents included;

- Nerol
- 2 different Eudesmols
- Citronellal
- Linalool
- Camphene / camphor
- Cadinene
- Terpinolene

- Arabinose
- Rhamnose
- Caffeic acid cinnamyl ester

A new ester (organic compound) in Asafoetida was isolated by *Abd El-Razek* and was reported in *'A new ester isolated from Ferula assa-foetida', pub. Biosci, Biotechol, Biochem; vol 71, issue 9, 2300-2303.*

Of all the plant's constituents and compounds, the sulphides, especially diasulphide $C_{11}H_{20}O_2S_2$, are primarily responsible for the plant's odour and flavour which are akin to strong garlic and onions. It is these sulphurous components that are used as perfume fixatives.

Research in Iran, *'Some like it pungent and vile. TRPA1 as a molecular target for the malodorous vinyl disulphides from asafoetida', by Shokoohinia Y et al, pub. Fitoterapia 2013 Oct; vol 90: 247-251/ Epub, NCBI 13.8.2013* found that activation of the TRPA1 molecule may be one of the actions underpinning ferula asafoetida, which due to its active sulphur bearing ingredients, has a mechanism similar to garlic.

As the plant ages, some of the essential oils convert into α pinene and β pinene and others are reduced an almost undetectable level.

The plant also contains a number of terpenes and lipid-soluble substances that have not been well characterised. Finally, there are caffeic acid, cinnamyl ester and sesquiterpene dienones (which have cytotoxic activity).

Significance of Ferulsinaic acid in ferula asafoetida

As we have seen, Ferulsinaic acid (FA) is a component of ferula asafoetida and its application in laboratory settings with different experiments on rats, guinea pigs or nematodes (*Caenorhabdtis elegans/ C. elegans)* has given promising results in the following examples;

- ✓ it appears to be remarkably potent at preventing protein glycosylation (modification)
- ✓ as well as normalising certain antioxidant enzymes, it is highly protective of the diabetic kidney. The ferulsinaic acid (FA) component in F. asafoetida can normalise antioxidant enzymes in diabetic kidney tissue. FA has also been found to reduce kidney weight in diabetic rats and is a potential drug for the prevention and therapy of diabetic nephropathy – *'Ferulsinaic acid attenuation of diabetic nephropathy ', Sayed AA, pub Eur Journ Clin Invest; vol 43, issue 1 Jan 2013 pages 56-63 (first published Oct 2012).* The prevention and therapy for DN by FA was also suggested in the paper *'Ferulsinaic acid attenuation of diabetic nephropathy', Sayed AA, Eur J. Clin Invest 2013, 43 (1): 56-63*
- ✓ it is possible for asafoetida, after daily ingestion for eight weeks, to increase the breakdown rates of

protein, fats and starches while accentuating sucrose absorption
- ✓ isolated Ferulsinaic acid has dose-dependently extended the mean lifespan and maximum lifespan of nematodes and also improved their heat stress. It had a therapeutic efficacy as an antioxidant with the possibility of its use as an antioxidant drug – *'Ferulsinaic acid attenuation of advanced glycation end products extends the life of Caenorhabdtis elegans' Sayed AA, J. Pharm Pharmacol 2011 Mar; 63 (3), 423 -428*
- ✓ asafoetida gum resin when used as a carminative, reduced contractions in the stomach of guinea pigs and this may mean that daily oral ingestion may reduce human flatulence with daily ingestion
- ✓ rats with high cholesterol, when given a supplement of 2% asafoetida were able to reduce their cholesterol levels in the blood (probably due to reducing absorption from the intestines)
- ✓ 200-400mg/kg of asafoetida gum extract was given to rats and at the higher dose there was better memory formation, although when compared to the reference drug rivastigmine at 5mg/kg it was weaker. Asafoetida could be complementary to existing anti-dementia therapies. It is thought that isolated compounds of the plant inhibit acetylcholinesterase (ac) and orally taking the gum extract inhibits ac activity in rat's brains. *(See report 'Evaluation of the effect of Ferula Asafoedita Linn. Gum extract on learning and memory in Wistar rats', Vijayalaksmi et al, Indian Journ. Pharmacol 2012 Jan; 44 (1): 82-7)*

✓ traditionally, ferula asafoetida has been recommended for various womens' reproductive ailments. A daily course (over 21 days) of oleoresin extract given to rats had anti-infertility results with pregnancy being prevented in 80% of rats; this result was not due to alterations in their oestrogen metabolism.

One paper on an experiment using rats to demonstrate the effects of asafoetida on relaxation was *'Antispasmodic and hypotensive effects of Ferula asafoetida gum extract'*, *Fatehi M, Farifteh F, Fatehi-Hassanabad Z, Journ. Ethnopharmacol. 2004;91 (2-3) 321-324.*

Another report using rats was *'The relaxant effect of essential oil and oleo-gum-resin of Ferula on isolated rat's ileum'*, *Bagheri S.M et al, pub Indian Journ. Nephrol, Nov-Dec 2016 26 (6): 419-422* concluded that asafoetida had a positive diuretic effect similar to Furosemide (a synthetic compound).

These experiments indicated that the isolated ferulsinaic acid used had a very low toxicity level and was in fact of such miniscule quantities that it doesn't practically matter. The basic gum extract didn't seem toxic at tested dosages.

Other research into the effects of asafoetida

Other research into the medicinal uses and benefits of asafoetida was carried out by clinicians and researchers at institutions in Iran, Saudi Arabia, India and Egypt. Countries where asafoetida is produced and/ or used significantly and where there is a long tradition of using the plant for medicinal, culinary and agricultural purposes.

A paper published in the *Research Journal of Recent Sciences (Vol 4 (IVC-2015), 16-22* (2015) *A Sultana, Asma K, K Rahman & S Rahman* www.isca, www.isca.me) studied the pharmacological activities of the oleo-gum-resin of ferula asafoetida as recorded elsewhere in international scientific papers about asafoetida. This activity was mainly in connection with rodents and other animals (with one exception, when groups of men were tested for its effects on libido and erectile dysfunction -see below) and the authors thought that the findings of these papers merited further studies of the effects of asafoetida on humans. The results indicated that asafoetida;

- o seemed to be a better treatment for anxiety disorders than the drug diazepam
- o exhibited a significant antinociceptive effect on chronic and acute pain in mice which most likely involves central opioid pathways and peripheral anti-inflammatory action
- o reduced the mean arterial blood pressure of a rat

- was as efficient as piperazine citrate in paralysing and then killing worms in a guinea pig's gastrointestinal tract
- had a therapeutic effect on asthma, probably because of its relaxation effect causing bronchodilation
- gave a notable improvement in libido and erectile function in men
- has an anti-obesity/fat lowering effect and can prevent liver steatosis in type 2 diabetic rats
- helped heal wounds including healing diabetic ulcers
- extracts from its leaf, stem and flower have proven antioxidant activity.

Effects of asafoetida on learning and memory function

An Iranian 2015 paper *'Influence of asafoetida on prevention and treatment of memory impairment induced by D-Galactose and NaNo2 in mice'* by Magheri and Dashti-R was published in the *American Journal of Alzheimer's Disease & Other Dementias (Vol.30(6) 607-612)*. This paper outlined the results of a study which was conducted on the learning and memory functions of mice and the effects on them of asafoetida.

The finding of this research was that chronic administration of asafoetida could prevent and treat learning and memory deficit in adult male mice in certain cases. It was also found that some of the key validated targets for Alzheimer's therapy are likely to be modulated by asafoetida. It is probable that any beneficial effects may be due to the presence of biologically active compounds in asafoetida such as contained in its sulphur constituent and sesquiterpene coumarins.

It is interesting that in the paper it was noted that in traditional Iranian medicine, asafoetida is introduced as a valuable remedy for nervous disorders.

Asafoetida and its anticancer activities

A published research paper, *'Evaluation of Ferula asafoetida for its anticancerous activities in different countries'* published in *the Journal of Pharmacognosy and Phytochemistry (2013; 2 (4): 74-76) by U Nigam and S Sachan* brings together the important link between the uses of this plant for medical and culinary purposes.

The authors identified the Ferula as a species which is used as a spice in many cuisines in many countries. Ferula has compounds which actively participate in the prevention of cancer and Ferula asafoetida was chosen from the 30 species of this plant.

They used World health organisation (WHO) statistics for the period 2008 – 2013 for their cancer rates (excluding non-melanoma) and the Central Intelligence Agency (CIA) library database for the population of a number of significant Asian countries during the same period.

This research showed that countries such as Afghanistan, India, Iran and Pakistan with a high usage and cultivation level of asafoetida when compared with countries such as Indonesia, Japan, Malaysia and Russia which had a much less common use of asafoetida and comparative population size had a much lower rate, and increase in incidence, of cancer.

Again, this research could be expanded to see if its conclusions could be replicated elsewhere in the world and if the use of this plant in its spice form could be used more to play a greater part in preventing cancer. If this is so, it could reduce the chances of the side effects which are normal in the existing conventional allopathic treatment of cancer.

Asafoetida and its action on foodborne bacterial and fungal organisms

The study *'Volatile oils from Ferula Asafoetida varieties and their antimicrobial activity', Divya K et al, pub LWT Food Science & Technology, Vol 59, issue 2 part 1, Dec 2014, pages 774 – 779* looked at two types (Pathani and Irani) of asafoetida and their efficacy against microbes associated with foodborne bacterial and fungal organisms. They concluded that the Pathani was an effective antibacterial agent e.g. against *Escherichia coli* and *Bacillus subtilis* and the

Irani type was an effective anti-fungicidal agent e.g. against *Penicillium chrysogenum* and *Aspergillus ochraceus*. This difference was due to their different major compounds.

Asafoedita as a mouthwash

A study *'The efficacy of Asafoetida (Ferula assafoetida oleo-gum resin) versus chlorhexidine gluconate mouthwash* (CHG) *on dental plaque and gingivitis: a randomised double-blind controlled trial'*, Hashemi M.S. et al, pub Eur. Journ. of int medicine, vol. 24 Aug 2019, 100929 looked at a trial on 126 patients. The results showed that the asafoetida mouthwash could be recommended as an efficient mouthwash and there were significant results in this group when compared to the group using the CHG mouthwash.

This study is an example of how modern scientific techniques are putting flesh on the old folklore traditions of using asafoetida.

Asafoetida and dyspepsia

A study *'Safety and Efficacy of Ferula asafoetida in Functional Dyspepsia: A Randomized, Double-Blinded, Placebo-Controlled Study'*, Mala K.N. et al, Pub 26.8.2018 in Evidence-based Complementary and Alternative Medicine, vol 2018 into the treatment of functional dyspepsia (indigestion/ impaired digestion) by using Ferula asafoetida oleo-gum resin showed encouraging results in patients, both remaining symptom free and having an improved quality of life.

Different international methods of medicinally using asafoetida

Asafoetida is used throughout the world for medicinal purposes and there are a number of different ways in different countries that this is done. These include;

- oral hot water extract of the plant in Afghanistan for hysteria, whooping cough and ulcers
- gum is chewed in Malaysia and Morocco
- hot water extract of the dried leaf and stem is taken orally in Brazil by males as an aphrodisiac
- in Saudi Arabia, dried gum is used for respiratory conditions such as asthma and bronchitis
- in India and Thailand, to aid digestion it is smeared on the abdomen in an alcohol or water tincture.

Asafoetida and Ayurvedic medicine

In Ayurvedic medicine bronchiectasis has hot energy counteracting Kapha (mucoid) and Vata (neurological) conditions. It is considered to be one of the best spices for balancing the *vata dosha* and this relieves flatulence and colic. When it aggravates P*itta* (fire digestive types*)* it enhances appetite, taste and digestion. According to Narayani's Indian Ayurvedic medicine book *'Materia Medica'*, asafoetida is both a valuable spice and condiment as well as serving as a valuable medical remedy. He lists a great number of ailments and conditions it can help and included in these are coughs, pneumonia and bronchitis in children and chronic bronchitis and asthma in adults.

There are many mentions of the medicinal use of asafoetida in Western and traditional Chinese medicine as well as in Ayurvedic medicine throughout the ages for many conditions. In all three of them it has been shown to be an effective remedy for the removal of worms and parasites It is thought that raw and unrefined asafoetida will cause nausea and vomiting.

In Ayurveda, it improves digestion through the prevention of ailments such as gas, flatulence, bloating and abdominal dissension. This improvement also leads to the prevention of the formation of excessive phlegm.

Although asafoetida is now rarely used in pharmaceutical preparations its use was mainly to stimulate the mucous membranes.

Middle East Unani/ Yunani medicine which is a Perso-Arabic homeopathic medical treatment based on the teachings of ancient Greek physicians such as Hippocrates and Galen, classifies asafoetida as Hot 4th degree and Dry to the 2nd degree.

Culinary uses

Asafoetida as a spice is used in a wide variety of food categories especially condiments and sauces and for pickling and is now readily available from the spice section of many food retailers. If used in cooking, asafoetida comes as a white powder. Although it has a very pungent smell, in cooked dishes it produces a flavour similar to that of leeks. Its pungent odour derives from sulphur compounds and its flavour becomes much milder and less pungent upon heating in oil or ghee (clarified butter). It helps to aid the digestion.

Asafoetida is a favourite spice in Indian cuisine especially for vegetarians. It is an ingredient in Indian lentil curries such as dal and is used in many vegetable dishes especially those based on potato and cauliflower. Kashmiri cuisine uses it in lamb/mutton dishes like Rogan Josh. It can even be mixed in a small amount with salt and eaten with raw salad. It can also be mixed with chili powder.

In Iranian cooking it is used for flavouring meatballs; in Afghanistan it helps in the preparation of dried meat.

Asafoetida is suitable for many fish dishes and some poppadoms are flavoured with it. It is important to stress again that because of its strong odour it has to be stored in an airtight container to stop tainting other foods nearby.

In Ayurvedic medicine, asafoetida is considered to be one of the best spices for balancing the *vata dosha* and this relieves flatulence and colic. When it aggravates *pitta* it enhances appetite, taste and digestion.

It is quite commonly used by Brahmins and Jains because onions and garlic are prohibited.

Other uses for asafoetida

Perfume

It can be occasionally used as a fixative and fragrance component in perfumery, especially rose bases and heavy oriental types.

Animals, fish and trees

In the USA its odour has strangely been found to be attractive to wolves and as a bait for catfish and pike. It has been known to be mixed with oil of anise and honey.

Along the South Indian coast, it is used to kill unwanted trees by boring a hole in the tree trunk and then filling the hole with it.

Pest control

It can be used as a light trap for moths after being mixed with sweet fruit jelly.

In Iran, which is one of the main centres of asafoetida production, there has been a great deal of research into its use as a natural pesticide. A paper *'Effect of fresh gum of asafoetida on the damage reduction of pomegranate fruit moth Ectomyelois ceratoniae in Shahreza City'* by M Kavianpour et al. was published in the *International Journal of Biosciences/ IJB vol5, No.5, p 86-91, 2014* which showed that with a treatment of fresh gum of asafoetida in a pomegranate orchard in the vicinity of Shahreza City (Istaphan province) there was better control of Carob moth (*Ect. ceraton*) damage, which leads to resulting rotten fruit than in a similar orchard which had not been treated. This is a good nonchemical means of pest treatment. This pest damages many other high value fruit commodities such as almonds, pistachios and dates in other regions of the world.

Also, in Iran, research has shown that asafoetida had been used to treat the green bean aphid which can be another devastating pest.

The History of asafoetida

Ancient history and the Middle Ages

In the 7th century BC, clay tablets in the library of **Assyria's King Assurbanipal** identified 250 vegetable drugs including asafoetida.

Since the 7th century, asafoetida has been used in Chinese medicine as a nerve stimulant in treating neurasthenia (fatigue, anxiety or listlessness). Traditional Chinese medicine also views it as entering the Liver, Spleen and Stomach channels. As well as stimulating the intestinal, nervous and respiratory systems it can be used for many specific conditions and imbalances including asthma and chronic bronchitis.

In traditional Indian medicine it was believed to stimulate the brain.

In the 6th century BC asafoetida was imported into Kirenaika/ Cyrenica (in today's Eastern coastal region of Libya) in North Africa from Kashmir in South Asia.

It was also brought to Mediterranean countries from Iran most notably by an expedition of **Alexander the Great (356BC – 323BC)** across the Hindu Kush mountains of Afghanistan.

It is believed that asafoetida superseded another herb which was a pungent fennel called silphium (also called lasar) of Cyrene/ Cyrenica (Kirenaika) which was more valuable and which became extinct during the **Roman Emperor Nero's** reign in the 1st century AD (54-68AD) because it was overharvested. The Romans used it as both a spice and for medicinal purposes and it was stored in jars together with pine nuts and used to flavour delicate dishes.

Disoscorides (40 – 90AD) was a Greek physician and pharmacologist, who was employed in the Roman army as a medic and who authored the *'De Materia Medica'* about herbal medicine and related substances, wrote about asafoetida in the first century AD.

Asafoetida was mentioned in Jewish literature such as the Misnah, which was a collection of Jewish oral traditions and the first major work of Rabbinic literature. Moses Ben Maimon who is better known as **Maimonides (1135-1204AD)** an eminent Spanish Jewish physician and philosopher also wrote about it (1170-1180AD) in the *Misneh Torah* which was a code of Jewish religious law.

Asafoetida, and its uses, was of great interest to many Arab and Islamic scientists, pharmacists and scholars including;

Avicenna (980-1037AD) who is also known as Ibn Sina or Abu Ali Sina was born in Bukhara, Uzbekistan and died in Hamadan, Iran was a very significant Persian writer, physician, astronomer, musical theorist and astronomer of the Islamic Golden Age. He was considered the father of early modern medicine and in his works included the effects of asafoetida on digestion.

Ibn al-Baitar (1197-1248 AD) an Andalusian Arab pharmacist, botanist, physician and scientist added knowledge about asafoetida together along with another 300-400 types of medicine to those known previously since antiquity.

Fakhr Al-Din Al- Razi (1150 – 1210 AD) a Sunni Moslem who was born in Rem (in modern Iran) and who died in Herat (in modern Afghanistan) was a famous theologian and philosopher. As well as being interested in medicine, physics, history and the law he described asafoetida's positive medicinal effects on the respiratory system (see *'Islamic Great Books of the World' ISBN 978-1-871031-687-6*).

Between the fall of the Roman Empire (476AD) until the 16th century AD, asafoetida was rare and it was considered mainly as a medicine. Many people thought that it would ruin cooking because of its smell, however some like **Garcia de Orta** *(1501-1568),* an eminent Portuguese Jewish physician and scholar, who wrote in 1563 an influential catalogue of Indian herbs and drugs, knew that it was used widely in India both for its culinary and medical properties. During the Italian Renaissance, asafoetida was used as part of the exorcism ritual and this use has been mirrored in the voodoo cultural tradition where it is used in magic spells for both good and bad.

Laurence's gardening and horticulture book written during the period known as the 'Age of Enlightenment'

Perhaps one of the most comprehensive historical books about asafoetida is the English gardening and agricultural book by **Rev. John Laurence** (1668-1732) which was *published in 1726* in the 'Age of Enlightenment' (which was a dominating intellectual and philosophical movement of ideas in Europe between the 17th and 19th centuries). This was entitled *'A new system of agriculture. Being a complete body of husbandry and gardening in all parts of them. Viz. husbandry in the field, and its several improvements'.* This long-overlooked book and its author deserve restoring to its rightful, high place in the annals of gardening and smallholding. Interestingly, knowing the interest in horticulture and gardening shown by Prince Charles, the current Prince of Wales, the book was dedicated to the then Princess of Wales!

This book is 456 pages long and it looks at asafoetida and its predecessor herbal plant silphium in detail in 17 of them (pages 384 – 400) such was recognised the importance of these two plants.

Much of Laurence's knowledge about asafoetida was the result of him visiting the Persian mountains in 1687 which was no mean feat at that time.

Apparently, at that time all the asafoetida used in Europe was brought there by the East India Company; it was grown In Persia (Now Iran). Laurence writes that it was mentioned ten years earlier in a book written by a German called **Kempfer**. Knowledge about asafoetida by Moslem scholars such as **Avicenna** and **Haltut** is recognised.

In Laurence's book, the structure of the plant (which was known as hungfeh); the soil it is best suited to; and the method of growing, harvesting and producing asafoetida and the plant's juice, which is called Hung in India, are all described in great detail. According to him one of its most striking features was its *'horrid, ungrateful smell of the Garlick Kind which is called by the Persians and Indians Hing and by the Europeans Asa Foetida'.*

Laurence wrote that Persia was its only native country of origin; certainly not Libya, Syria, Cyrene or China.

In Persia there were only two locations where it was best grown – the fields & mountains around Heraat and the range of mountains in the province of Laar. Apparently, goats became fat if they fed on the plant's leaves!

As it took four seasons work to prepare and harvest the plant, the workers ascertained beforehand what the demand for the asa would be so that their work would not be in vain; a sign of market forces at work several hundred years ago!

Even then it was known that the application of seeds of the plant could be used to kill worms at the base of any plant or tree. In Laar, its medicinal properties were known and it was used for digestive conditions, colic and to improve the appetite.

Laurence even speculated on the possibility of introducing the plant into Britain but it seems that two great obstacles to be overcome were the need for the great summer heat the plant needs and the possibility that fat sheep would gorge themselves on its enticing leaves so reducing production levels. Perhaps, with today's climate change or global warming, things may change!

Since the nineteenth century

The shock of its sulphurous smell was once thought to calm hysteria and in the days of the American Wild West in the 19th century asafoetida was mixed with other strong spices as a cure for alcoholism.

Asafoetida was mentioned in many medicinal books including *King's American Dispensatory* (first published 1854) and the *Indian Materia Medica* by K M Nadkani (first published 1908).

In the form of an alcohol or water tincture (a medical solution) asafoetida was used as a topical treatment for abdominal injuries in the West in the 18th & 19th centuries. A Canadian, Alexis St. Martin suffered a severe abdominal injury from a shooting accident which perforated his right lung and stomach and shattered several ribs. He was treated by **William Beaumont**, an American army surgeon and pioneering digestive researcher, who when the wounds had healed inserted different foods into an open fistula into St Martin's stomach to record the results. One insertion, three times daily, was a combination of wine mixed with diluted muriatic acid and 30-40 drops of tincture of asafoetida. This concoction helped the wound to heal.

In the USA in the 19th century the use of asafoetida was promoted by 'Eclectic' doctors especially for the women's condition 'hysteria' which according to Freud is the root of the word 'hysterectomy'. The Eclectics were one of the three major medical sects then in the USA (the others being the' Regulars' and the' Homeopaths'). These sects disagreed about how to treat patients and their conditions and each sect thought that their treatments were the most effective and scientific type of practice.

Because asafoetida was thought to be helpful in treating respiratory conditions such as asthma, bronchitis and whooping cough it was used during the 1919 Spanish influenza pandemic.

Although asafoetida is a plant with significant international economic, medicinal, culinary and cultural importance significance the author found that in the UK and Ireland there were only two major botanical gardens where it is being grown (at December 2019). Some other botanical gardens only had exhibits in their herbarium in pressed form but had grown it in the past.

The two botanical gardens were;

- ✓ the world renowned, centuries old Chelsea Physic Garden, London (www.chelseaphysicgarden.co.uk) whose Director kindly informed me that the plant is represented in three of their collections – in the Future Medicine Bed, in the Garden of World Medicine: India bed, and in the Dicotyledon order bed. Seed is collected and sown in the Autumn; although the plant is hardy, it is replanted from time to time. The Garden is part of the Index Seminum which is the International Botanic Gardens seed exchange programme. Seeds are shared with other botanic gardens under an established convention and if there is sufficient seed of ferula this could be made available on this programme for other botanic gardens to apply for
- ✓ at the Millennium Seed Bank, Wakehurst Place kept by the Royal Botanic Gardens (RBG) there

are specimens of seed of Ferula foetida, one accession collected in Kazakhstan and the other collected in the Kyrgyz Republic. Wakehurst has germinated plants. At the RBG Kew, London there are some plants which were grown from seed collected in Tajikistan. This information was kindly supplied by K. Pennick, the Wakehurst Place Librarian.

The Objectives of this chapter were:

1. to allow the reader to see in detail how the asafoetida essential oil vapour can be used in an easy to prepare self-treatment session(s) for a respiratory condition like bronchiectasis
2. to give the reader an overview of the importance, and different uses of, asafoetida a plant which has been used (for medical, culinary and other purposes), researched and written about since antiquity.

Suggested further reading

'The Illustrated Encyclopaedia of Essential Oils' by Julia Lawless, published by Element books (ISBN 1-85230-661-0)

'Description of asafoetida plants (Narthex asafoetida, Falconer) which have recently borne flowers and fruit in the Royal Botanic Garden of Edinburgh' 1860 by John Hutton Balfour. Published by Neill & Co (ASIN B0008781VS)

'A new system of agriculture. Being a complete body of husbandry and gardening in all parts of them. Viz. husbandry in the field, and its several improvements by Rev. John Laurence, published in 1726 (ISBN 9 781170 788837)

Publications by the UK charity 'Plants for a Future', whose website (www.pfaf.org) lists the cultivation and edible and medicinal value of ferula asafoetida. Email address: admin@pfaf.org

CHAPTER 4: USING THE PULMONARIA (LUNGWORT) PLANT

The Aims of this Chapter are;

1. To describe how I use the pulmonaria (lungwort) plant in a beneficial way to help my bronchiectasis
2. To explain why pulmonaria is such a valuable plant in helping cope with bronchiectasis and to give information, including research, about it.

Introduction

Having learnt, after hospital diagnosis, that I suffered from bronchiectasis which is a long-term respiratory condition I decided to see if I could use any natural plant products to help manage the worst symptoms of this debilitating condition. By taking this course of action, which was an alternative to conventional, (mainly) antibiotic drug therapy, I hoped to avoid the possible negative side effects of these drugs and also reduce the risks to me, associated with the growing resistance of bacteria to antibiotics which is one of the greatest and growing dangers facing modern allopathic (science based conventional Western medicine) medicine.

In the last chapter, I explained how I chanced upon the essential oil derived from the (ferula) asafoetida plant and the way that it had helped me through the inhalation of its vapours which is a very unusual way of self-treatment.

The second type of plant I assimilated into my own self-help programme is pulmonaria; I have had a long interest in them and had always admired them elsewhere when I was working as a professional landscape gardener in London.

I now grow about ten different pulmonaria species and cultivars, predominantly *Pulmonaria* officinalis, in my own small semi- shady back garden. I have found that all the varieties of pulmonaria ('*P*'), whether having plain, silvery or spotted leaves, I grow give an excellent drink; if anything, the silvery leaved species e.g. *P. 'Blake's Silver'* or *P. 'Calverley Gem'* seem to give the better results.

The drink they produce is refreshing, pleasant and cleansing and its taste is similar to that of Earl Grey tea but without its (bergamot) scent. It leaves no after-taste and is unlike any of the many other herbal or fruit teas that I have tried. I don't add any sugar, sweeteners, milk, honey or lemon to the 'tea' but you could do that if you prefer a different taste. It can be drunk either hot or cold.

What is pulmonaria?

The plant genus (family) pulmonaria is mainly known in the UK as lungwort, which is its common (synonym) name. Pulmonaria is a member of the Boraginaceae family (all plant families have the suffix 'aceae') and is a relative of many other plants including borage, comfrey, forget-me-not and viper's bugloss.

Although pulmonaria grow in the wild, especially in shady woodland locations, it is a relatively easy, low growing perennial and ornamental, plant to cultivate. Most of them are semi - evergreen but a few can be completely deciduous. It has been very popular for both its flowers and often-variegated leaves.

Its species (a group of plants that share a genetic heritage similar to each other & are capable of interbreeding with each other to produce fertile offspring) and cultivars (varieties which have been bred by man for desirable features such as flower size or colour or variegated foliage) are well known to many gardeners.

The development and appearance of pulmonaria leaves

In the garden (and also in the wild), there will be both new and developed leaves which can be picked when the plant is actively growing, usually between late February and the end of autumn (the period will vary depending on location, weather and environment). When picking leaves, please remember not to over - pick as this may threaten the plant's survival. Also, **never dig up plants in the wild** as they may not live after being moved to a different growing environment such as in a garden.

The leaves of pulmonaria *(P)* species and cultivars range in shape from being lanceolate (pointed) e.g. *P. affinis* through to being oval e.g. *P. officinalis*. They also have a range of green shades with an overlaid pattern of spots or smudges of cream, white or silvery white in a pattern which resemble either a diseased lung or the tissue inside a lung. However, some are green without a pattern e.g. *P. 'Blue Ensign'* or are silvery white e.g. *P. Majesté.* All leaves, with some exceptions (e.g. *P. mollis*), are rough and covered with minute, protective hairs which are usually rough or bristly (which act as a deterrent to slugs, snails, deer and rodents).

Reasons, and options, for using pulmonaria

Knowing that this plant's leaves and flower stems had been used for healing purposes for respiratory, and other, ailments since ancient times throughout the world I thought I would see if it could help me with my bronchiectasis.

Although it is the leaves and flowering stems which are used for medicinal purposes, I decided to use only its leaves and not its rhizome, roots, flowers, or flower stem.

There were three options about how to use the plant's leaves and these were;

1. to eat the leaves raw. As the leaf's surfaces are usually covered in hairs it is not really pleasant that they be eaten raw such as in a salad; preferably the leaves should be used fresh in soups, stews or used as a vegetable. The spring and summer are the best times to do this

2. to use it in a tincture (when combined with alcohol) or capsule form. As I am not a qualified aromatherapist, herbalist or druggist I didn't think this option was practical for me
3. to use the leaves in a drink similar to a herbal tea; they can either be picked and immediately infused fresh or dried and changed into 'tea leaves' for use at a later time.

The third option of drinking pulmonaria in a 'tea' form was the most appealing to me, but I did also discover an associated method of eating its leaves (after being drunk as a tea).

How I use pulmonaria leaves

Picking and preparing the leaves

Once a plant has a reasonable number of new developed leaves, these can be picked by hand or cut off with a pair of scissors. Even though additional leaves will continue to grow, please take care not to denude the plant completely.

Being keen to try to follow an organic food diet as much as possible, no commercially produced pesticides or herbicides are used on any of the plants (including pulmonaria) in my garden.

If there is any dirt or insects on the leaves these need to washed off. Bear in mind the fine hairs on the underside of the leaves; gloves could be worn but this precaution is not usually necessary -it is unlikely that any skin irritation will be caused, but please take care when handling this plant, especially if you find that you have an allergy to it.

Once the leaves are ready, I pick and tear them into small pieces. I also remove and discard the conspicuous central, thicker, midrib vein which runs up from the base to the apex of the leaf. If any leaves have developed mildew – don't use them and dispose of them (preferably in a compost bin or in the 'green' recycling collection).

Making fresh pulmonaria tea

I put approximately two or three teaspoons of pieces of the freshly picked leaves (or one or two teaspoons full when using already prepared dried leaves), into an infuser and this is placed and left steeping/brewing in a cup of boiling water for a few minutes.

There will be a gradual change in the water's colour which is due to its absorption of the properties of the leaves. The length of time the infuser is in the cup will vary depending on the preferred strength of drink which is required; practice will make perfect. After boiling the leaves, the hairs on the leaves are no longer felt.

After all the liquid has been drained from the infuser, the used 'tea' leaves can be retained to make a second or perhaps, even third drink (the second is usually stronger; with the third drink having a weaker colour and taste than the second drink). The number of drinks will depend on the initial number/ amount of leaves being boiled.

Unlike many other teas it has an advantage in that it doesn't leave a stain mark on the inside surface of a cup (so making washing- up easier) or staining on the teeth after use.

Homemade pulmonaria tea leaves

As well as using picked fresh leaves in an infused pulmonaria 'tea', the leaves can be turned into dried 'tea' leaves for future use by baking them in an oven. The oven is preheated and then the fresh leaves are broken up into pieces and spread out on a baking tray. As a guide, the leaves are baked/ dried for 1½ to 2 hours at 40-50°C (104-122°F). Please experiment with timings and temperatures as all ovens have different power settings and so behave differently. You could start out making a small batch to get the hang of the process with waste being minimised if things go wrong.

It is important that all moisture is removed from the leaves and once ready, the baked pulmonaria 'tea' leaves are removed from the oven and allowed to cool. They should then be put into an airtight container and stored in a cupboard or other dark place.

Using commercially prepared pulmonaria tea leaves

An alternative to using your own pulmonaria leaves, or to augment your own supply, is to buy ready prepared, processed and packed pulmonaria 'tea' leaves. These purchased leaves should be preferably organic, free from preservatives, colourings and bulking material and should be stored in an airtight container in a cupboard. The pulmonaria tea I have bought was commercially produced in Spain; I am sure that sources from other countries are available. Unfortunately, there was little information on the packaging about the tea's constituents.

These purchased tea leaves are infused as a drink in the same way as homemade pulmonaria 'tea' as described above. Again, a drink's strength depends on the amount of leaves to be infused; one or two heaped teaspoons (approximately one gramme) should suffice for 2/3 cups. After they have lost their strength the used leaves can be added to other food dishes (see below). Purchased leaves can be especially invaluable in the winter if the supply of your own home-grown pulmonaria 'tea' leaves runs out.

Some other people leave the leaves (fresh or prepared) infusing for up to fifteen minutes in 150 ml of boiling water before drinking them, the problem with this is that the tea is likely to go cold before being drunk! You might like to try the tea cold, as a refreshing drink, in the summer if the weather is hot.

Eating the used tea leaves

After the leaves have been used as a tea for the last time, I drain and remove them from the infuser and add them to any of the food dishes I am then eating e.g. breakfast cereal, porridge, soup, yogurt or on toast with jam, honey or marmalade etc.

Food for the dog?

On a light cautionary note, my dearly departed, very intelligent 13 years old pet black Labrador- cross dog Tizzy must have seen that I use pulmonaria leaves for drinking and eating because she often ate the leaves straight off the plants in my garden before I could harvest them! She didn't come to any harm, must have had great lungs and certainly didn't have any breathing problems!! However, it was very galling that she regurgitated the digested leaves on my lawn after eating them -it is probable that the hairs on the underside of the leaves irritated her throat.

My new Jack Russell terrier dog also likes to drink pulmonaria tea when he thinks that I am not looking. The moral of these two stories seems to be - keep an eye on any of your loveable potential four- legged pet pulmonaria leaves or tea bandits!!!

Drinking pulmonaria tea as part of a balanced fluid intake

Pulmonaria tea, whether made from freshly picked leaves or from dried leaves, as well as having a pleasant taste, is gentle and has benefits such as being astringent (one meaning being the restriction of fluids such as checking the discharge of mucus). This is a natural product and should not be adulterated in any way. It can be drunk like an ordinary tea or other herbal tea.

As well as drinking pulmonaria tea I also drink other beverages including water, decaffeinated tea and decaffeinated coffee and a small amount of alcohol. I would suggest that all consumers of pulmonaria tea (and other herbal teas) combine and vary their intake of pulmonaria tea with other beverages which will give a balanced fluid intake and has a health significance as will be explained later in this chapter.

The principal constituents, and their actions, of pulmonaria

Pulmonaria leaves and stems have a high mucilage (liquid) content which makes it especially useful for the treatment of chest conditions especially chronic bronchitis, bronchiectasis and chronic coughs.

The plant's other constituents include; alkaloids, tannins, saponins (any of a group of plant glycosides that produce a soapy foam in water), allantoin, silicic acid and calcium carbonate (found in the hairy bristles), bioflavonoids (quercetin and kaempferol), ascorbic acid (vitamin C) and micro amounts of mineral salts including manganese, iron and copper.

Pulmonaria's constituents have a number of actions and these are;

- astringency (contracts tissue, dries up secretions and stops bleeding)
- demulcent (soothes and protects the mucous membranes and relieves irritation),
- diaphoretic (induces or increases perspiration),
- diuretic (stimulates the elimination of water by increasing the production and flow of urine),
- emollient (soothes and softens the skin)
- expectorant (stimulates the expulsion of phlegm/sputum from the respiratory tract).

Saponins

The saponins are a class of natural plant phytochemical chemical compounds which are also found in other plant species such as most vegetables and herbs including peas, beans and soybeans. They have anti-inflammatory and immune boosting properties and antibacterial effects and their specific actions include;

- reducing total and LDL (bad) cholesterol levels whilst not affecting HDL (good) cholesterol levels
- killing of disease- causing bacteria
- scavenging oxidative stress

- inhibiting tumour growth
- improving lipid metabolism
- helping to treat and prevent obesity
- encouraging sneezing (which helps clear the nose, nasal and facial sinuses).

How can pulmonaria work medicinally?

In a pulmonaria 'tea', the leaves' expectorancy powers can relieve respiratory congestion and ease a sore throat. This type of tea is likely to have a high phenolic content and antioxidant properties (see research paper *'Polyphenols and antioxidant capacity of Bulgarian medicinal plants'* by *Ivanova D, et al, pub. Journ. Ethnopharmacology 2005 Jan 4; 96 (1-2): 145-150, pub online 17.11.2004'*. Of the 21 Bulgarian plants screened, only seven, including *P. officianalis*, had high phenolics (chemical compounds which are associated with a decreased risk of chronic disease) content and antioxidant properties (compounds which can indirectly inhibit the release of damaging free radicals in cells). These seven were considered to be a rich source of phenolics compounds and /or water-soluble antioxidants when compared with other plants which had been studied.

Pulmonaria is effective against harmful organisms that affect lung and chest function due mainly to its high level of flavonoid glycosides (another name for specific types of antioxidants which are crucial for supporting organ's health and function) together with the properties of its saponins.

The pulmonaria's allantoin content is anti-inflammatory and soothing and its vitamin C is good for treating colds and other ailments.

Pyrrholizidine alkaloids (PAs)

Having read in Masha Bennett's excellent book 'Pulmonarias' (details at the end of this chapter) the section on the presence of natural compounds called Pyrrolizidine Alkaloids (PAs) in some plants of the Boraginaceae family and their toxicity if consumed in sufficient quantities I thought that it would be important for safety's sake to do some detective work and look into this subject in more detail. This is why I have listed so many different research papers and reports about PAs, and their findings concerning pulmonaria, which have been produced in different countries.

I must say that I haven't had any health ill effects from drinking pulmonaria tea and it should be remembered that the strength of the pulmonaria contained in a first cup of tea is reduced if used in a subsequent or even third cup. My views on the matter are expanded later in this chapter.

PAs are nitrogen- containing compounds which are natural toxins when biosynthesised by plants as a defence against herbivores. Approximately 6,000 plant species worldwide which represents 3% of all flowering plants may contain PAs and to date, an estimate of approximately 600 different PA structures is known. PAs are present in more than twelve plant families, in particular Boraginaceae, Asteraceae and Fabaceae.

The PA content depends on a number of factors e.g. species, plant origin, age, harvest and extraction procedures. Because of their different structures and characteristics, not all PAs are toxic to humans. The biggest risk is posed by 1,2-unsaturated PAs. Any PA toxins are most commonly concentrated in the seeds, roots and rhizomes and much less than in the leaves, flowers and flowering stems of a plant. This can vary between species however.

There has naturally been a lot of interest in PAs and how food (including honey; dairy produce especially milk; meat and eggs), animal feed, herbs, teas and herbal teas which contain them can affect humans and animals. The presence of many of the PAs identified in foodstuffs were found to be due to contamination during production and processing.

These types of alkaloids are also well known for their wide range of pharmacological properties which can be exploited in drug discovery programmes. Referring to the report *'Pyrrolizidine Alkaloids: Chemistry, Pharmacology, Toxicology and Food Safety'* by *Moreira R. et al* published in *'International Journal of Molecular Sciences'* (5.6.2018) para 3.2.1 quoted for instance that the alkaloid usaramine was analysed concerning its ability to inhibit biofilm formation in

Staphylococcus epidermis and *Pseudomonal aeruginosa*. While there was no effect on *P. aeruginosa* there was a 50% prevention in biofilm formation by *S. epidermis*. This report also included details of PAs being used for research into anti-microbial and anti-inflammatory activity (3.2.1 & 2), anti-cancer activity (3.2.3), anti-HIV activity (3.2.4), AchE enzyme inhibitors (3.2.5) and miscellaneous conditions such as NSAID induced gastric ulcers (3.2.6). No reports of cancers found in humans as a direct consequence of PA consumption were found (4.2).

In Moreira's report there is a detailed table of medicinal species containing PA. There are twenty-three species in the Boraginaceae family listed, but Pulmonaria is not included in the list. This list was compiled based on the work (1995 and 2000) of Prof E Roeder (see below).

The chemistry of PAs has been researched worldwide and a significant contribution was made by *Prof. Dr. E Röeder* (a noted pharmalogical professor emeritus at Friedrichs – Wilhelms University, Bonn, Germany) and his findings were published in *"Pharmazie" 50 (2) (1995) pages 83-98*. He based his conclusions on the research work of *(i) Roeder E, Britz-Kirstgen, R, Unpublished results (1984) and (ii) Leuthy. J, et al: Pharm. Acta HeR. -9, 141 (1984)*.

Prof. Roeder looked at a number of families of plants, including Boraginaceae, which has about 150 genera and 2,500 species, of which pulmonaria is a member.

In the genera and species of this vast family it was only *P. officinalis* which did not contain PAs (report's section 4). However, in his list (section 4.1.1 – 4.1.10) of twelve medicinal plants in this family, including common bugloss, borage, garden heliotrope and common comfrey, which contained PAs, no species of pulmonaria was included.

In the report *'Safety Issues Affecting Herbs: Pyrrolizidine Alkaloids'* (www.itmonline.org/arts/pas.htm) *by Dharmananda S.*, the expert status of Prof. Roeder in studying PAs in plants was acknowledged. In table 1 of his report entitled *'Plants that contain Pyrrolizidine Alkaloids'* it was stated 'that the PA content of *P. officinalis* is questionable'. As well as ingesting PAs directly from plants, it can also be consumed from honey collected by bees which have visited PA containing plants and also from milk or eggs from animals which have consumed PA-containing plants. He summarised human toxic reaction to different herbs and of the small number described (less than 15), the main problems lay with the use of comfrey in (herbal infusions), heliotropium and coltsfoot. Pulmonaria was not mentioned in this respect. He also questioned the potential carcinogenic effects on humans of long-term use of herbal preparations containing PAs for many months or years. This report also questioned the effects of deeming any amount of PA in herbal products as a contraindication as this would restrict many herbal products as PAs have been found in members of ten plant families other than the three families listed earlier in this chapter.

The British Ecological Society has written in its journal *'Biological Flora of the British Isles: Pulmonaria officinalis'* by *Meeus S. et al* published 20.8.2013 that the roots (but not the leaves) contain PAs.

A report by *Luthy L. et al* in his report *'Pyrrolizidine alkaloids in medicinal plants of Boraginaceal: Borago officinalis and Pulmonaria officinalis'* pub *in Pharm Acta Helv. 1984; 59 (9-10): 242-6* stated that 'no PAs could be detected in several samples of the drug Pulmonaria officianalis L.

Another piece of research into pulmonaria and PAs was carried out by *Haberer W. et al*, and his report *'Pyrrolizidine alkaloids in Pulmonaria obscura'* was pub in *Planta Med. 68: 480-482 (2002)*. He studied and analysed, using more sensitive testing techniques, the rhizomes, roots, leaves and inflorescences of *P. obscura* plants and their content in PAs. The total PA concentrations in the rhizomes and roots was between 0.026 and 0.158mg/g dry weight; in the leaves and inflorescences only trace amounts (below 0.4 ng/mg dry weight) of PAs could be detected.

A book by *Plumlee K.H. published by Mosby Inc* and publicised in *Clinical Veterinary Toxicology (2004)* contained a table (25-8) listing plants that have been associated with PA poisoning. In the Boraginaceae family, of the thirteen named plants pulmonaria was not included with respect to animals and humans.

In Germany, the BfR (Federal Institute for Risk Assessment, www.bfr.bund.de) issued a detailed report (BfR Opinion 018/ 2013 of 5.7.2013) which included an analysis of 221 samples of commercially available teas, herbal teas and herbal drugs for their PA content. The assessment of possible health risks used the international MOE (Margin of Exposure) standard. It found that 'for consumers, both adults and children, with an average consumption of herbal tea and tea who do not favour a specific variety health impairment due to chronic intake of PAs is improbable' (page 1). 'If people frequently drink large quantities of herbal tea and tea, risk of health impairment can be reduced by varying and diversifying the choice of food' (page 1.)

In this BfR report no mention was made of any risk of drinking tea made from pulmonaria. This was unlike the risk associated with other plants (see its page 6) such as Heliotrope, common groundsel or Alpine ragwort (*Senecio alpinus*).

The efsa (European Food Standard Safety Authority) produced a report '*Scientific Opinion on Pyrrolizidine alkaloids in food and feed*' pub *EFSA Journal 2011; 9 (11): 2406* and it concluded that in humans there was some concern for toddlers and children who are high consumers of honey and generally a low risk of PA poisoning in livestock and companion animals in the EU. Although the increasing use of herbal dietary supplements was mentioned, especially those with PAs which are used in traditional Chinese medicine no mention was made of any pulmonaria species.

In the article *'Pyrrolizidine and tropane alkaloids in teas and herbal teas peppermint, rooibos and chamomile in the Israeli market* by Shimshoni J. et al published in *Food Additives & Contaminants: Part A (2015)* looked at dehydro (chemical compounds which have lost one or more hydrogen atoms) PAs and tropane alkaloids (TA) which are prevalent in the Bor*ginaceae and* other plant families. They get into the food chain, including teas and herbal teas, often by contamination at harvesting and production levels. Dehydro PAs were found in both teas and medicinal herbs and the levels varied between type and these were often different to those based on samples used in European tests. Tea using pulmonaria leaves was not mentioned in this article.

The European Medicines Agency (EMA) produced on 31 May 2016 a *'Public statement on contamination of herbal medicinal products/ traditional medicinal products with pyrrolizidine alkaloids'*. This statement was accepted by the European Union's Committee on Herbal Medicinal Products (HMPC). *The statement* contained a number of relevant statements, including about health problems in humans caused by high doses of 1,2 -unsaturated PAs. These health problems were based on only the few documented cases which have been recorded and it concluded that a small daily intake of PAs from herbal medicinal products will not constitute a risk for development of HSOS liver damage (section 2.1). Although the human intake of PAs through food and herbal products has been constant over the last decades (or longer); the incidence of hemangiosarcoma liver (HL) damage caused by PAs has been very low and is in fact very rare. To put the risk level into perspective, Zochetti in 2001 concluded that based on studies in Sweden, UK, USA and Norway the cases were 0.5-2.5 cases per 10,000,000 individuals and of these 20/25% cases were associated with other causes. Other research has concluded that the causes are unknown (section 2.4). Of the 10 herbal ingredients requiring routine controls Pulmonaria was not included (section 6.2).

Another interesting study into PAs, *'Pyrrolizidine Alkaloids in Food', 'Risk Assessment Study Report No.56'* was published by the Hong Kong government's Centre for Food Safety (www.cfs.gov.uk) in January 2017. In this report, over 100 food samples tested included individual 1,2-unsaturated PAs and these included duck eggs, yoghurts, cheeses, honey, tea and herbal tea beverages. Common teas contained relatively low PA concentrations while some tested 'specific teas' (such as rooibos tea, verbena tea and peppermint tea) and 'dried spices' (such as cumin seed, oregano and tarragon) had relatively higher levels of PAs. <u>The study advised the public to maintain a balanced and varied diet including a wide variety of fruit and vegetables so as to avoid excessive exposure to any contaminants from a small range of food items (study's Para 13).</u>

A review *'Diversity of Pyrrolizidine Alkaloids in the Boraginaceae Structures, Distribution and Biological*

Properties' by *El-Shazly A. and Wink M.* published in *'Diversity' April 2014, 6 (2), 188-282* reported the available information (up to 2014) about the status of PAs in the Boraginaceae family of plants. This review contained a list of species containing PAs and of the 218 listed only *P. obscura* of the Pulmonaria was named (this was sourced from the report of Haberer, details shown above). A second list showed that *P.obscura* contains the alkaloids 7-Acetylintermedine and Lycopsamine (source, Haberer) – this species is used in some vermouth drinks.

Looking at the situation regarding professional herbal practitioners, a list of certain PA- bearing herbs which should not be prescribed for internal use (*PA– generating herbs – BHMA-EHPTA working list, 8 August 2016*) was issued by the EHPTA (European Herbal and Traditional Medicine Practitioners Association, (www.ehtpa.eu). On this list, neither *P.officinalis* or any other pulmonaria species were named.

Interestingly, the position of the BHMA (British Herbal Medicine Association)/ EHTPA is that all parts of *P. officinalis* are likely to contain unsaturated PAs and until further research is carried out, the use of it as a herbal medicine is not recommended due to the potential for long-term (20-30 years) health issues such as liver damage and liver cancer.

At the moment, there seems to be a divergence of international views, conclusion and recommendations contained in the existing research and reports which have been carried out into plants and their PAs and their effects on public health. On the whole, with a few significant exceptions, it would seem that the best course is to follow a varied and balanced fluid intake to minimise any minutely possible risk.

The Author's view about pulmonaria and PAs

After studying all the above (and other) studies, reports and views into, and about, pulmonaria and PAs and considering any minimal risk linked to the amount and strength of the pulmonaria tea I drink and because it forms only one part of my balanced fluid intake I feel that it is a safe thing for me to continue doing. I feel that the present ongoing benefits to my respiratory health outweigh any unproven risks to my long- term (20-30 years) health.

Obviously, it is up to each individual to make his/ her own decision whether to drink pulmonaria tea or not. if anyone suffers an adverse reaction to drinking tea made from pulmonaria leaves (or from any other source) they should stop using it.

The traditional medical uses of pulmonaria

- The parts of the pulmonaria plant which have been traditionally used medicinally are the leaves and the flowering stems. These are best harvested in the spring and early summer and are then dried and made into infusions and extracts

- The leaves are used in herbal medicine, in an infusion to soothe respiratory conditions such as bronchitis, chronic coughing and whooping cough. Its anti-inflammatory and astringent properties help it treat diarrhoea and other gastrointestinal conditions. The success of pulmonaria may be due to the fact that it contains natural antibiotics which act against bacteria

- Externally, it is used in compresses and as a bath preparation for wounds and skin disorders such as eczema, haemorrhoids, varicose veins and burns. Success may be due to the silica and allantoin in the plant. The leaves' astringency explains why it helps staunch bleeding

- Lungwort is believed by flower essence practitioners to open psychic airways and to loosen the blockage of repressed emotions

- In astronomy, lungwort is associated with the Pisces star sign.

Background information about pulmonaria

Pulmonaria 'aliases'/ synonyms

The name pulmonaria/ lungwort is derived from the Latin word 'pulmo' meaning lung and the ending 'wort' which simply means plant (other examples are Ragwort, Mugwort and Soapwort).

'officinalis' as in *pulmonaria officinalis* is a Medieval Latin epithet (to put on to or to add to) denoting mainly plants (or organisms) with uses in medicine and herbalism and it is the second term of a two- part botanical name.

In Germany and Sweden, the common name also refers to the lungs ('lungenkraut' and 'lungört' respectively); in Easter European languages, the name relates more to honey e.g. 'miodunka' in Polish and' medunitza' in Russian

It has a number of synonym names including; 'Soldiers and Sailors', 'Bloody Butcher', 'Boys and Girls', 'Adam and Eve', 'Spotted Dog', 'Joseph and Mary', 'Bethlehem Sage', 'Our Lady's Milk Drops', 'Jerusalem Cowslip', 'Jerusalem Sage' and 'Virgin Mary's honeysuckle'. Another name is 'Mary's Tears' so called because the white spots on the leaves resemble her tears and the changing colours of the flowers from blue to red represent blue eyes becoming reddened through crying. The biblical connection is obvious.

Where does pulmonaria grow?

Pulmonaria grows widespread throughout Europe from England, Spain and Portugal in the West to Siberia in the East, from Italy and Greece in the South and to Sweden in the North. It is most common in central Europe and came to the UK from Europe and Eurasia.

The majority of pulmonaria growing wild are found in shady or partially shaded places such as different types of deciduous woodland (in particular in the understory of broadleaved mixed open woods rich in hornbeam, beech and oak), conifer and yew woodland, shrub and the banks of rivers and streams. It is necessary to regularly open the tree canopy to maintain viable populations in the long term.

They often grow at higher altitudes probably because of their cooler climates in Slovakia, Romania, Germany, Austria and Italy. Some pulmonaria however grow in open meadows and on rocky slopes. They are hardy plants and can tolerate minimum winter temperatures down to -29°C (-20.2°F).

Estimates about the number of pulmonaria species that are native to Europe and the UK and which grow in the wild vary between ten and eighteen. It has only relatively recently that they have become native to the British Isles. They are widespread, predominantly in the south of the UK and are sparser in Scotland, Ireland and the North of England.

According to the 2019 UK Hardy Plant Society (HPS) book *'Pulmonarias'* over 275 pulmonaria species and cultivars are listed which have either been cultivated or happened by chance. This number can fluctuate because some become lost and others are continually being introduced by plant breeders and others. It is most of these which are available to grow in a garden setting in the UK.

Pulmonarias thrive in shady, semi shady and damp parts of the garden and prefer these conditions to a dry and sunny spot although some can tolerate a sunnier aspect e.g. *P. 'Cambridge Blue'* and the *P. officinalis Cambridge Blue Group.*

They like chalky ground as well as a clay soil. The soil should be moist as well as having good drainage. It can be grown in large pots, in which the compost is kept moist and in which its creeping roots are allowed to spread.

It is a good plant to grow (the opposite to hostas) if you don't want a lot of slugs and snails in your garden. These little creatures are probably deterred by the plant's hairy exterior!

Pulmonaria growth

Depending on its variety, it grows from 15 – 40 cms (6 – 16 ins) high with a spread of 45 – 60 cms (18 – 24 ins). It has creeping rhizomes which help it spread and all some parts of the plant are stiffly hairy.

Pulmonaria flowers

Pulmonaria is attractive in the spring because it has tiny pretty flowers which can be any of the following colours - red, blue, purple, violet, white or a mixture of these colours and their shades.

Pulmonaria is a deciduous plant/ herb which is often considered to be just a decorative spring perennial plant valued for its distinctive patterned leaves as much as for its tiny, pretty five petaled (corolla) flowers.

The colours of the flowers can change during the season after fertilisation, for example from pink in bud to a variety of shades of blue as the flower ages. The colour change is associated with a complex change in acidity with a higher acidity/ low pH in a young pink or red flower to a lower acidity/ higher pH as the flower ages with a resultant change to blue. This colour change mechanism in the flower is a signal to the pollinators about when best to visit the plant - when the nectar level is high before it falls thereafter. At times, a pulmonaria plant can bear flowers which are both pink and blue.

Pulmonaria insect pollination

Pulmonaria are pollinated by insects, and are especially attractive to early foraging solitary bees who are attracted to its early production of nectar and also later in the year to bumble bees and honey bees. Bees prefer the blue flowers which are borne by many pulmonaria. Often in the spring it is in flower before most other plants and *P. officinalis* is one of the earliest pulmonaria to flower.

The culinary uses of pulmonaria

Raw pulmonaria leaves can be added to salads, soups and stews; they are low in fibre and are best picked when young before their protective hairs have become harder. The leaves are also palatable when cooked as a vegetable although they are quite bland in taste and become slimy if cooked for too long.

Pulmonaria 'obscura' has been one of the herbal and botanical ingredients used for flavouring the Vermouth alcoholic drink (other plants used in this respect have included chamomile, coriander, gentian, saffron, juniper and wormwood).

In medieval times pulmonaria was often used in stews and savoury dishes. Pulmonaria saccharata in particular has been used as a spice.

The history of pulmonaria

Between 1348 and 1350 the pandemic 'Black Death' or Bubonic Plague swept across Europe killing many millions including an estimated 4.2 million in England. Lungwort was used to try to cure the plague when It was used together with wormwood (Artemisia absinthium).

In Europe in the 16th and 17th centuries, lungwort became used more to treat lung and breast conditions. In England in the 17th century, lungwort was called 'Jerusalem cowslip' and was used for asthma and bronchial problems.

On a darker side of the middle ages, in parts of Europe lungwort was used as a proof to see if a person was a witch. By wearing lungwort this could be a protection against witches and evil beings.

Taxa of lungwort was mentioned in British horticultural books by; **John Parkinson** (1629), **John Gerard** (1633) and **Phillip Miller** (1768).

In Britain, pulmonaria was first cultivated around the end of the 16th century and recorded in the wild from 1793 (in Kent and SE London). It was grown for both medicinal and garden ornamental use and in the USA, it was found in their first botanical garden near Philadelphia which was established by **John Bartram**, a Quaker in 1728.

Selective pulmonaria breeding really developed in the twentieth century.

At the moment in the wild, pulmonaria is under threat in many parts of Europe (including in Suffolk with *P.obscura*/ Suffolk lungwort) and it is important to help protect it by regular opening of the tree canopy and increasing gene flow between plant populations.

Pulmonaria obscura Dumort

This a species of Pulmonaria which is very rare in the wild in the United Kingdom, although it is widespread within Europe. It merits mention, because it crops up in much of the medical research listed previously in this chapter. It has unspotted leaves and a learned article was written about the species '*Pulmonaria obscura Dumort*' by *C.R. Burkinshaw and M.N. Sandford* published in '*Watsonia21; 169-178 (1996) (www.wats21p169.pdf)*

It has the synonym 'Suffolk Pulmonaria' because it was first mentioned as growing wild in that county in 1832. It is now only found in three Suffolk wooded areas (Burgate Wood, Stubbings Wood and Gitting Wood) which are all privately owned. It was first listed in the RHS Plant finder directory in 1992 and last listed therein in 2006. There is great concern about its conservation (see species of Conservation Concern List, Natural History Museum, London).

As we have seen, Pulmonaria obscura has been used as a flavouring in vermouth, an alcoholic drink.

Notable botanists and pulmonaria

Theophrastus Paracelsus (1493- 1541) listed lungwort in his book *'Doctrine of Signatures'.* He thought that plants resembling certain human physical attributes were beneficial to the body part to be treated. So, as Goldenrod was thought of as a cure for jaundice because of its yellow colour, so lungwort could treat lung problems because of the spotted lunglike pattern on its leaves.

Giambattista Della Porta (1535 – 1615) was a botanist, polymath and founder of the world's first scientific society. in *'Phytognomica'* his book (1588) on the *Doctrine*, it is clear that that the plant called pulmonaria with hairy leaves like bugloss, spotted white with purple flowers, commonly called 'cynoglossa' (with a woodcut which could be *P.*

officinalis) indicated its use for ulcerated lungs, spitting blood, shortness of breath and asthma.

It is listed and shown as a woodcut in the '*A niewe Herball*' (1578) by **Henry Lyte** (1529(?) – 1607), the English botanist. He called it Sage of Jerusalem and says it is of 'no particular use in physicke, but is much used in meates and salads with eggs, as is also Cowslippes and Primroses, whereunto in temperature it is much alike'.

Nicolas Culpepper (1616 – 1654) English herbalist, botanist, physician and astrologer wrote in 1653 in his book the *'Complete Herbal'* that he found many sorts of lunguewort and that they 'help infirmities of the lungues, as hoarseness, coughs, wheezing, shortness of breath etc'.

Matthais de Lobel (1538 – 1616) and **Pierre Pena** were French botany students who met at the Garden of Medicinal Plants (now the Chelsea Physic Garden), London. They co-wrote the *'Stirpium Adversaria Nova'* botanical tome in 1570 and it included a Latin description of pulmonaria. It translates as 'PULMONARIA spotted, Borage -leaved, flowers like Primula veris -Cowslips – purple'. They added that women mix the leaves with a little broth and make it into an omelette for lung disorders and to strengthen the heart. The importance of this volume is reflected in the auction price in 1997of a first edition reached US$ 50,600!

In 1576 Lobel calls it Maculosa Pulmonaria and depicted a white flowered form in a good woodcut.

Lobel was so highly regarded that the plant Lobelia Cardinalis was named after him!!

John Gerard (1545 – 1612) English herbalist and botanist published his *'Illustrated Herball'* in 1597. He used the same pulmonaria woodcut as Lobel and calls it Pulmonatia foliis Echii, Buglosse Cowslips with red flowers. Also, a woodcut of a narrow leaved plant described as Pulmonaria masculosa, Spotted Cowslips of Jerusalem with red, blue and purple flowers and says 'the leaves are to be used among pot-herbs and the roots are also thought to be good against the infirmities of ulcers of the lungs...'

Sourcing new pulmonaria plants

If the reader wants a guide to the best pulmonaria to use, a list of *P. officinalis* plants will be found at the end of this chapter. The Royal Horticultural Society's (www.rhs.org.uk) annual reference directory *'The Plant Finder'* lists nurseries which can supply pulmonaria and other plants. The 2020 edition became available in April 2020. Many garden centres, local nurseries and plant sales are other sources for pulmonaria plants.

The Objectives of this chapter were;

1. **to allow the reader to see in detail how the pulmonaria/lungwort plant has been used to treat my bronchiectasis**
2. **to give the reader an overview of the importance of, and different uses for,**

pulmonaria/ lungwort, a plant which has been used, researched and written about since antiquity.

Suggested further reading

'Pulmonarias and the Borage Family', *by Masha Bennett, 2003, Published by B T Batsford, (ISBN 0 7134 8732 1)*

'Pulmonarias', by Margaret Stone & Jennifer Hewitt, 2nd edition 2019, Published by the HPS Hardy Plant Society (www.hardy-plant.org.uk) a UK registered charity, (ISBN 978-0-901687-32-6)

'Discovering the Folklore of Plants', by Margaret Baker, Published by Shire publishers, (ISBN 9 78 074780178-8).

A list of Pulmonaria officinalis plants' names

'Alba'; 'Bamberg'; Blue Mist'/ 'Blue Moon'/ 'Bowles's Blue'; The Cambridge Blue group including 'Cambridge Blue' and 15 other plants; 'Coral'; 'Marjorie Lawley'; Stillingfleet Gran'; White Wings'; 'Wuppertal'.

'Sissinghurst White' was originally assigned to the P. officinalis species but is now described as hybrid and P. Rubra is now not assigned to the officinalis species.

CHAPTER 5: IMPROVING BREATHING

The Aims of this Chapter are;

1. **to describe how I tried to improve my breathing to help, and reduce the effects of, my bronchiectasis**
2. **to explain why improved breathing is a valuable way to improve the respiratory system in particular and the body's physical, mental and emotional condition in general**
3. **to have a brief introduction to some of the different methods and systems which are available to help improve people's breathing.**

Introduction

Although it seems to be stating the obvious, without natural breath, everybody will lose the ability and means to function and the result will be that death will ensue. The importance of breathing is demonstrated by the estimation that bodies can go without food for several weeks; without water for several days; but only three minutes without drawing breath before the average human suffers brain damage and about ten minutes before death. Exceptions are free divers who train themselves to hold their breath for extended periods (possibly over twenty minutes) and people who follow certain meditational forms of religion/ discipline.

As breathing (or ventilation) which moves gas in and out of the lungs will affect the whole body if it is not done correctly then the mind & body will not be able to perform to its full potential. With better breathing, performance will improve and life will feel better. While this is true for bronchiectasis (and other respiratory conditions) sufferers, it is also a significantly important thing for sportspeople, singers, musicians, actors, students of all ages studying for examinations and many others to help them in their activities and achieve their goals.

Having too little oxygen in the body can lead to symptoms including dizziness, confusion, headaches and in extreme cases hypoxaemia, when there is not enough oxygen in the blood to effectively nourish the cells, tissues and organs. Hypoxaemia can be acute (happening suddenly) due to something such as a blocked airway or chronic (over a long time) due to a lung condition, asthma or anaemia.

If the quality and quantity of breathing is reduced, perhaps because someone has damaged airways or is possibly due to a chronic lung condition such as bronchiectasis, then this will have a serious negative effect on the overall health and wellbeing of the sufferer.

If the effects of this reduced level of affected breathing can be improved, this should lead to a better health outcome for the person affected. This can be achieved by both improving breathing and implementing some other health and lifestyle changes including;

- ✓ doing more exercise, as this helps muscles become more efficient in receiving and storing oxygen
- ✓ giving up smoking (or not starting in the first place)
- ✓ limiting exposure to pollutants e.g. when doing housework chores, use natural products and open windows to increase ventilation
- ✓ in the UK use the 'CleanSpace' air pollution mobile phone app to see pollution levels in your area and plan journeys to avoid them (similar apps will be available in other countries)
- ✓ walking down quieter streets with less traffic pollution and walk on the inside of the pavement to reduce exposure to harmful fumes by as much as a third
- ✓ closing vents and windows in your car when stuck in traffic
- ✓ wearing a face mask/ covering if cycling, walking or simply being in crowded or indoor places such as public transport or bars. This has become mandatory in some instances with the COVID -19 pandemic
- ✓ planting evergreen hedges, shrubs and suitable trees in your garden to help them absorb CO_2 from the atmosphere; try to persuade your local council to do the same on the roadside and also reduce unnecessary tree felling. Those which are planted should shed little or no pollen into the atmosphere
- ✓ trying to add certain foods to your diet which are thought to help the lungs e.g. garlic, ginger, turmeric, onions, dark fruit berries, nuts, broccoli and chilli.

Some people however can over- breathe and the signs of this include;

❖ breathing totally through the mouth rather than in through the nose and out through the mouth
❖ needing to take large breaths before talking
❖ loud breathing when at rest
❖ breathing through the upper chest rather than deeper from the diaphragm.

How I tried to improve my breathing

The main purposes of improving my breathing were;

1. to increase the amount of oxygen taken in during inhalation
2. to expel more stale air from the lungs during exhalation
3. to use the lungs more efficiently.

Before deciding which of the many breathing methods which are available would best meet my needs, I thought that I should analyse my existing method of breathing to see what simple changes could be made immediately.

In this book's foreword you may recall that when I attended a breathing clinic as a schoolboy, mention was made by my respiratory specialist that I breathed incorrectly with an open mouth during both inhalation and exhalation. **I therefore decided to concentrate on breathing-in through my nose and breathing out through my slightly open (with pursed lips) mouth.**

As well as always previously breathing- in through my open mouth and very often breathing- out through my mouth, I realised that I was a shallow- breather during both my inhalation and exhalation and this meant that I was not fully utilising the lobal capacity of both my lungs.

Hopefully with deeper breathing, accumulated carbon dioxide, which is a cause of yawning, will be reduced and that yawning will consequently be reduced.

I could choose my breathing method from any of the numerous breathing systems and methods which are available, some details of which are included later in this chapter. These can be sourced through the internet, books and magazines and in the local reference library.

They include yoga breathing poses; the Pilates breathing and posture method; the Alexander technique; the Buteyko breathing method which originated in Russia; and the 'Active Cycle of Breathing Technique' (ACBT) which is taught to patients by specialist- chartered physiotherapists in the UK's NHS.

The ACBT technique is often allied to the teaching of gravity assisted positioning/ postural drainage (PD) which uses different body positions, mainly when lying sideways at an angle on a bed, to help the drainage of secretions from targeted areas of the lungs and to help increase the air movement or ventilation to different parts of the lungs.

I chose to adopt and practice a simple diaphragmatic breathing pattern because;

- ✓ of its simplicity and is easy to do and practice
- ✓ it minimises my own mobility issues
- ✓ it avoids complications in adjusting the position of my bed if doing PD.

My pattern consists of;

- ➤ either standing upright or sitting in a supportive chair
- ➤ placing the palm of one hand on the chest with the other palm placed on the abdomen/ lower stomach midway between the ribs
- ➤ the shoulders and upper chest should be relaxed throughout both the breath- in/ inhalation (when the chest expands) and breath- out/ exhalation (when the chest relaxes).

Inhalation is through the nose, and the back of the ribcage is accordingly expanded like two balloons. The inhaled oxygen spreads right down to the lower lobes of the lungs. The hand lying on the abdomen will rise first and that on the chest will hardly move. There will be a period of holding/ retaining the breath, and then exhalation will follow with the body movements being the opposite to those experienced with inhalation.

My recommended, simple breathing method is as follows;

1. breathe- in/ inhale through the nose (with the mouth closed) for about two seconds (2)
2. retain the inhaled breath for about four seconds (4)
3. breathe-out/ exhale fully for about four seconds with the mouth slightly open, with pursed lips, as if you are blowing out a candle on a birthday cake – it should be like a breathy, seashore sound (4).

This is a ratio of 2:4:4 (breathe-in: hold breath: breathe-out). It is best if the abdominal muscles are contracted/ tightened during exhalation. The lungs will be emptied more than when normal, quiet breathing takes place. **I call my system: 'The Breathing Cycle Ratio Method'.**

It is more economical to increase ventilation (moving gas in and out of the lungs through inspiration and expiration) by breathing slower and deeper. This may feel strange at first because the normal rhythmic breathing pattern is active inspiration (I) and passive expiration (E) at an I:E ratio of approximately 1:2.

I have added the element of retaining held breath. Although I have never studied yoga, I found that the retention of breath is similar to the practice in that discipline which is described near the end of this chapter.

I am mindful that many people have their own method of breathing, with different rates and depth of breathing and these variables may have to be changed for improvement.

To start with I would recommend that two breathing cycles are done normally with the in- breath through the nose with the mouth closed and then the out-breath done through the open mouth with pursed lips. The cycles can be increased gradually probably up to six times per session

After a number of inhalations and exhalations cycles with the 2:4:4 ratio this can then, with practice, be increased gradually up to 5:10:10 or above; the number of repetitions being those which are comfortable for you.

I would suggest that this breathing Method is done in periods, progressing up to six times daily. The length of each individual cycle can be varied within a session to make it more interesting and can be a fun challenge to you. Once you get good at the doing the Method, challenge others to a competition with you!

If a group of people (e.g. a sports team or orchestra members) are practising the Method together in person or by video link a safe competitive element can be incorporated to see if/ by how much progression is being made.

As deep breathing and physical exercise/ activity are the two main methods of clearing lung secretions naturally, it is expected that secretions will be loosened and these can be coughed up and cleared (preferably on to a handy tissue which is then hygienically disposed of).

If the deep breathing of my Method causes the chest to become sore, reduce the intensity or number of repetitions but keep to the principles of the method and try to do it daily.

As well as deciding on the procedure of my Method I also decided that I would need to try to strengthen my willpower to continue with it even though I was using my health club facilities (or exercising at home when the club was shut during the Covid-19 lockdown), out walking my dogs daily, or doing the gardening.

Without regular attention to detail and keeping to my planned breathing programme I was less likely to improve my breathing.

As well as doing my own breathing Method I supplemented this by using a simple to use and cheap inspiratory muscle training machine which is designed to increase the strength and durability of the respiratory muscles. The one I chose was the 'Ultrabreathe adjustable exerciser (www.ultrabreathe.com) but other different models are available and these can be viewed on internet shopping sites. Other customer comments, on internet shopping sites, about different aids is helpful and could save you money.

Knowing the importance of measuring any results from doing work to improve my breathing I found it interesting and reassuring to find that when doing a

'Control Pause' breathing test (which was devised by Dr Konstantin Buteyko) the result showed a significant improvement. I went from 'having health problems' to having 'satisfactory health'.

In addition, I found it very reassuring that my recent hospital pre-op spirometry test result showed that my lung age was ten years below my actual age. This finding, when combined with my metabolic age test, indicates I am doing something right with my own practical health philosophy including using my Breathing Cycle Ratio Method.

How the respiratory system works and why it is so important to improve it

In chapter one we looked in detail at the form and function of the various structures involved in the respiratory process. Breathing (or ventilation) is the process whereby inhaled air passes into and out of the lungs to allow the blood to take up oxygen and nitric oxide gas molecules (through the walls of the lung's alveoli) and dispose of carbon dioxide, which is produced by cell activity, from the venous blood (again, through the walls of the alveoli). This process is known as the Gas Exchange.

Perhaps with the importance of Nitric Oxide (NO) in helping breathing, specifically by nasal breathers, which is emphasised later in this chapter this gas should be included in the constituents which comprise the Gas Exchange.

While the process of breathing is in essence something most people usually take for granted it is only mainly when problems occur and the respiratory system doesn't work properly that thought has to be given to improving matters. This is certainly (or should be) the case when people suffer with chronic breathing or lung conditions such as bronchiectasis, bronchitis, COPD, asthma; cystic fibrosis (which is caused by an inherited genetic defect); or unusual conditions such as the 'Pickwickian syndrome' which is due to having excess weight or 'Obesity Hypoventilation Syndrome', symptoms of which are disordered sleep and sleep apnoea.

There are three methods of breathing which people do (mostly) without thinking and these are;

1. only breathing through the open mouth
2. partial nasal breathing, with the in- breath being done through the nose and the out- breath through the open mouth
3. total nasal breathing, with both the in- breaths and out- breaths through the nose.

Mouth- only respiration gives lower levels of oxygen (O_2), carbon dioxide (CO_2) and nitric oxide (NO) within the body's cells. It is thought that mouth- only breathing can be a leading cause of mortality in severely sick patients with chronic conditions. Is it any co-incidence that the early morning hours of 4-7am have the highest death rates due to coronary-artery spasms, anginas, strokes and asthma attacks?

There have been a number of studies which have studied;

- the CO2 - related biochemical effects of mouth respiration
- the benefits of nose breathing, in delivering NO to lungs, blood and cells.

Carbon dioxide (CO2)- related effects of mouth respiration

CO2 is not a toxic waste gas and it is stored in the 'dead space' inside the nose, throat, bronchi and lungs. Possibly the most significant of these 'dead spaces' are those found within the lungs, bronchi and trachea.

These anatomical dead spaces in the air passages contain air which doesn't reach the alveoli during respiration. The alveolar dead space is the sum of the volumes of the alveoli which have little or no blood flowing through their adjacent pulmonary capillaries and where no gas exchange can take place.

The total physiological dead space is a combination of anatomical dead space and alveolar dead space and while it is minimal in healthy lungs it is increased with most lung disease such as bronchiectasis.

The CO2 can be used during inhalations to help other parts of the body via the alveoli of the lungs. With mouth respiration, 'dead spaces' decrease because the nose is not used as part of the breathing route. Air exchange for mouth- breathing is stronger because inhaled air goes directly to the alveoli. This reduces alveolar CO_2 and arterial blood CO_2 concentrations. This effect does not happen with nose breathing.

CO_2 is a waste gas produced when carbon combines with oxygen and is associated with energy making processes in the body by the mitochondria within cells.

Mouth-breathing provides less resistance for respiratory muscles than nasal breathing because the route for mouth-breathing is shorter and has a greater cross-sectional area.

The report *'An assessment of nasal functions in control of breathing'* by Tanaka et al, 1 October 1988 *published* in *Journal of Applied Physiology, Vol.65 No.44* found many negative biomechanical effects of mouth breathing when related to CO_2 including;

- reduced oxygenation of the whole body
- constriction of blood vessels due to CO_2 deficiency
- reduced oxygenation of cells and tissues of all vital organs
- anxiety, stress, addictions, sleeping problems and negative emotions
- slouching and muscular stress
- biomechanical stress due to cold, dry air entering the lungs (so take care if out running or doing activities, such as gardening or DIY, outside in the winter months – possibly cover your mouth with a scarf)
- biomechanical stress due to dirty air (viruses, bacteria, harmful chemicals etc) entering the lungs

- possible infections due to the absence of the self-immunisation effect
- pathological effects due to suppressed nitric oxide utilisation including the decreased destruction of malignant cells in the lung's alveoli.

Nitric Oxide (NO) – Benefits and importance of nose- breathing oxygen delivery to the lungs and body

Nitric Oxide (NO) is a significant and important molecular gas which is produced by cellular organelles, including mitochondria, in all body tissues including in the nasal passages and the sinuses but not in the mouth. We earlier looked briefly at its significance in chapter one.

The NO molecules which are continuously being produced in the nasal cavity can therefore be utilised and directly passed to the lungs with breathing- in through the nose unlike breathing - in through the mouth.

NO inhaled through nasal inhalation is significant to respiration because it;

- increases blood flow through the lungs and boosts oxygen levels in blood
- dilates constricted pulmonary arteries and increases blood flow in the lungs
- relaxes smooth muscle in the airways -trachea and bronchioles and makes it easier to breathe

- enables red blood cell haemoglobin to extract more oxygen and pass it into general circulation

Other functions of NO include;

- destruction of viruses and parasites in the airways and lungs (and elsewhere in the body) by inactivating their respiratory chain enzymes
- vasodilation of arteries and arterioles which regulates blood flow
- promotes blood flow to all organs
- inhibits effects of inflammation in blood vessels
- has hormonal effects, in that it influences secretion of hormones, including adrenaline, pancreatic enzymes and gonadotropin- releasing hormone, from several glands
- affects transmission of neural signals. Memory, sleeping, learning, feeling pain processes are only possible in the presence of NO.

Other medical treatments utilising Nitric Oxide

Nitric Oxide (NO) dilates, by relaxing arteries' smooth muscle, the blood vessels of heart patients so reducing their blood pressure and heart rate; this gives them a better chance of surviving a heart attack.

NO is given to 'blue babies' with persistent pulmonary hypertension of the newborn to increase their oxygen intake (turns them 'pink') and has been successful in saving many lives.

NO is undergoing trials in the USA to see if it will help treat patients with the COVID-19 virus.

NO is the principal mediator of penile erection and sexual arousal which led to the development of Sildenafil/ Viagra which works by enhancing NO.

The importance of NO was recognised in the joint award of the 1998 Nobel Prize in Physiology or Medicine to Furchgott R., Ignarro L. and Murad F. *'For their Discoveries Concerning Nitric Oxide as a signalling molecule in the Cardiovascular System'.*

The benefits of cleaning, humidifying and warming inhaled air when nose/ nasal breathing

Nasal passages are able to humidify, clean and warm incoming air flow due to a protective thin layer of mucus. The mucus traps approximately 98-99% of unwanted bacteria, viruses, dust particles and other objects.

Athletes and asthmatics should live and train mostly and probably better with nose breathing. Nose breathing should bring better aerobic results. Certainly however, great care should be taken when doing strenuous exercise or activities outside during cold weather, mainly in the winter when deep breathing with cold air entering the lungs is not to be recommended and a protective face covering should be worn.

The body's natural self- immunisation when breathing – in through the nose

It is thought that a thin protective layer of mucus moves naturally as a long carpet from the sinuses, bronchi and other internal surfaces towards the stomach. Accordingly, if nasal breathing takes place, any objects trapped by the mucus are discharged into the stomach where gastrointestinal enzymes and hydrochloric acid either kill or severely weaken bacteria, viruses and fungi.

At a later stage of the digestive system, the damaged pathogens can penetrate from the small intestine into the blood system but there they cannot do much harm or cause infections. This natural process is mimicked when vaccines with dead or wakened bacteria or viruses are injected thereby teaching and strengthening our immune response to these pathogens. Nasal breathing is important to create conditions for natural self- immunisation.

The importance of different sleeping positions

Because the action of breathing is not spread evenly around the different parts of the lung(s) the lying position is very relevant to everyone, especially those suffering with a respiratory condition.

The lung's alveoli in the lower regions can be squashed by the weight of the lungs, which are heavy with blood, above and around them. A horizontal, supine (face-up) position is good although this is not the case with children, obese people and those on ventilators.

Side-lying is even better and the lower lung will have increased breathing ability and when supported, the diaphragm will be free from abdominal pressure. Compared to a supine position there is an increased lung volume, improved gas exchange and a reduction in the work of breathing.

Deep, shallow and slow breathing

Deep breathing has several advantages over shallow breathing and these include;

- the quadrupling of Work of Breathing (WOB) which can include the oxygen consumed by respiratory muscles
- lung ventilation is encouraged and diffusion (equilibrium of gases between air and blood, so leading to easier movement of gas to the blood's haemoglobin) is increased
- anatomical and alveolar dead spaces (which when summated is the physiological dead space) in the lungs is reduced. Anatomical dead space is the area in the trachea, bronchi and air passages containing air that doesn't reach the lung's alveoli during respiration. Alveolar dead space is their total volumes which have little or no blood flowing through their adjacent capillaries. This is important for people with lung conditions such as

bronchiectasis who should be breathing deeper rather than faster
- shallow breathing is inefficient because the same air is going in and out more often.

Deep breathing exercise advanced guidelines

Advanced deep breathing exercises aimed at increasing lung volume should be;

1. done in cycles of 3-4 breaths which will help maximise effort in each breath; dizziness from over- breathing is avoided; and shoulder tension is minimised
2. a few seconds break to allow a person to resume a relaxed approach
3. performed at least 10 times per hour when awake as this will encourage alveoli to stay inflated
4. the in-breath should be comfortable and slow, through the nose and out through the mouth
5. the in- breath should be deep into the abdomen to work the whole lung rather than a shallow breath which only utilises the upper portion of the lung
6. after the end of the out-breath a little extra air can be expelled by blowing out (through pursed lips).

Different breathing methods

I have already explained earlier in this chapter how I devised and use my own Breathing Cycle Ratio Method. In the rest of this chapter, I have outlined in more detail the different systems of improving breathing to the one I use which can be tried by bronchiectasis (and other respiratory) sufferers to help their condition. It could be that relief will be found after experimenting with them and then using what gives each individual the best results.

Whilst the description of each system is necessarily brief, more details about them can be found on internet search engines, in text books and magazines, in the local library or better still by directly contacting a specialist respiratory physiotherapist, a relevant organisation/ charity or an accredited local teacher/ instructor.

As well as working on improving someone's physical state, better breathing should also help the emotional side and some will even say the spiritual side of someone's wellbeing.

Breathing exercises if done correctly and regularly should relax the body naturally and this will make breathing easier. Relaxation is a recurring theme with each method of breathing exercise system.

The Active Cycle of Breathing Technique (ACBT)

This technique is taught to patients by most respiratory chartered physiotherapists they see in the NHS and is a patient self- help method they use after they have received instruction from the therapist.

It is often used together with Postural Drainage (PD) if this appropriate for the patient. The aim of the PD technique is to use gravity, when the patient is lying in different positions on a bed, to help clear excess mucus/ secretions, from the lungs, which are associated with conditions such as bronchiectasis, COPD and cystic fibrosis. Mucus and excess secretions can increase problems with infections and inflammation which can block smaller airways.

ACBT is a sequence which is made up with a combination of;

- ✓ gentle breathing control which helps relax you and your upper chest and airways
- ✓ deep breathing which loosens secretions
- ✓ 'huffing' or forced breaths-out, is done by exhaling through an open mouth and throat, at medium and high volume and for different lengths of time; this helps secretions to move into a better position to be cleared and coughed out.

The different parts of ACBT are carried out in cycles and the technique can be done in a sitting position or in the Postural Drainage (PD) positions. ACBT is repeated several times daily, more often when there is an infection. ACBT should be completed when the chest feels clear or the patient tires. It is important not to 'huff' too forcefully. Complete the full cycle and end with relaxed abdominal breathing.

Autogenic drainage (AD)

Autogenic drainage (AD) is also taught to patients by specially trained respiratory physiotherapists for a patient's self -use later.

AD produces a high airflow in the bronchi. Secretions which are not accessible using other physiotherapy techniques such as PD and massage are cleared from the small peripheral airways through to the larger central airways by a three- phased breathing pattern ranging from a low volume to a medium and then finally a large volume breath. Overall, AD will gradually increase lung volumes.

AD can be done daily and takes between 30 – 45 minutes. It improves the saturation of haemoglobin with oxygen (SATs) and in research into the use of AD with COPD patients it is as effective in mucus clearance as ACBT. It seems reasonable to assume that this will also be the case with bronchiectasis sufferers.

Bubble-positive expiratory pressure (bubble-PEP) type of airway clearance technique (ACT)

An interesting small study with great potential was conducted in Australia which showed that this the form of ACT (bubble-PEP) could be effective in helping clearing sputum from people with stable bronchiectasis and could be considered as an alternative method of sputum clearance technique to ACBT. This study *'Bubble-positive expiratory pressure device and sputum clearance in bronchiectasis: A randomised cross-over study'* by *Santos M.D. et al.*, was published in the journal *'Physiotherapy Research International'* on 29.2.2020. It was found that while there was no significant difference in the produced wet weight of sputum between bubble-PEP and ACBT during a 30- minutes intervention, sputum wet weight was significantly greater with bubble-PEP than ACBT after a period of 60 minutes after the intervention. A control group showed less sputum weight production than either those using ACBT or bubble-PEP.

An advantage of the bubble-PEP device is that it can be easily made by a therapist and is cost effective being made using easily available and disposable materials (a small bottle containing a small amount of water and a connecting tube). It can be used by children and adults; children (and some adults) can enjoy playing games blowing bubbles in the bottle.

Postural Drainage (PD)

Postural Drainage (PD) is done with someone lying on the edge of the bed in several different body positions using gravity assistance to help secretions drain from particular targeted parts of the lung(s). It also helps to increase the movement or ventilation to those parts. Side-lying helps the lower lung's breathing augmented by twice that of the upper part.

Specific PD positions are recommended for the lung condition being treated, as well as the affected part of the lung(s) which are being targeted. As with breathing techniques, the patient's physiotherapist will advise which positions should be used.

Often, the head is at a different level than the chest in tipped - up positions. If these positions are uncomfortable, they may make the patient breathless. It is also possible that this position might increase food reflux from the stomach. If either of these results happen, the physiotherapist will suggest some options for the patient such as doing an airway clearance in the sitting position.

To reduce the risk of stomach content reflux, PD should be done at least one hour after eating food. An additional aid may be an electric, adjustable bed which raises at either the head or lower end.

Diaphragmatic Breathing (DB)

The diaphragm is located at the base of the lungs and it, together with the abdominal muscles help breathing, together they powerfully empty most of the inhaled air. Diaphragmatic breathing can strengthen the diaphragm and help the breathing become more efficient with more oxygen reaching the body's cells.

Proper, deep breathing engages the pelvic floor and the body's core muscles as well as being a lifelong remedy for stress. By strengthening the pelvic floor this will help with the problem of incontinence suffered predominantly by women (especially pre and postnatally) which is both embarrassing and deters many sufferers from exercising.

Diaphragmatic breathing (DB) also works the transversus abdominis muscles of the tummy muscles or inner core which helps keep us strong throughout our lives.

DB can be done in several ways, including

Method one;

1. inhale through the nose and imagine the back of the ribcage expanding like two balloons so that the inhaled oxygen is spread down to the lungs' lower lobes
2. exhale fully through the mouth like you are blowing out the candles on a cake with the lungs completely emptied
3. engage the pelvic floor by lifting it and drawing in the belly button and then inhale and release
4. This should be done by gradually working up to six inhales and exhales daily.

Method two;

1. lie down with a pillow under the head and another under the knees
2. place one hand over the upper chest and the other below the rib cage over the stomach
3. inhale through the nose; keep the upper hand still and breathe into the stomach so the hand on it can be felt moving out
4. exhale through the mouth; the hand on the chest should again be still and the hand on the stomach

should now move towards you. Contract the abdominal muscles to push out all the air
5. take slow and steady inhales and this should be repeated several times daily

There are advanced methods of practising this method and for those with limited mobility it can be done while sitting in a chair or standing. Overall, this is a good way of reducing stress levels. After a while the hand positions can be dispensed with.

Other physiotherapy - taught breathing methods

Although the Active Cycle of Breathing (ACBT) technique is the most common method taught by UK physiotherapists, other techniques taught or used include;

- positive expiratory pressure (PEP)
- oscillating positive expiratory pressure (OPEP), using devices such as the 'Flutter' and the 'Acapella'
- autogenic drainage (AD), details on page 213
- intermittent positive pressure breathing (IPPB)
- high frequency chest wall oscillation (HFCWO)
- intrapulmonary percussive ventilation (IPV)
- intermittent positive pressure breathing (IPPB).

Minimising the effects of breathlessness

Many people who suffer from bronchiectasis, and other lung conditions, suffer from a shortness of breath which affects them adversely and restricts their activities. It is useful if they can minimise potential problems that breathlessness can cause and ways of doing this include;

- ✓ plan ahead and pace yourself
- ✓ avoid periods of overactivity followed by underactivity – be constant
- ✓ use breathing exercises and co-ordinate breathing with activities
- ✓ lift properly and safely, know your limitations and minimise twisting movements
- ✓ have a clean home with good ventilation
- ✓ sit while doing tasks and activities – it uses less energy than when standing
- ✓ minimise arm exertion especially above chest height e.g. rest elbows on a worktop
- ✓ maintain good posture and don't compress the lungs
- ✓ consider sleeping in different positions to help reduce pressure on the lungs
- ✓ use good body movement and avoid (where possible) bending, reaching and twisting
- ✓ use supports and equipment such as 'grabbers', an electric toothbrush and have casters under furniture
- ✓ reduce maintenance tasks in gardens e. g reduce cutting a lawn
- ✓ use a fan to improve air flow
- ✓ rest if necessary during exertion and avoid physical activities for one hour after meals

- ✓ get help from friends and outside organisations/ agencies e.g. buy delivered prepared meals or employ a house cleaning person etc
- ✓ improved breathing helps relaxation and reduces stress.

Specific ways to reduce breathlessness

People who suffer from breathlessness can benefit greatly from a system of desensitisation to the fear that doing activity with resulting breathlessness is in itself is harmful. This process is probably best done by a therapist who has built up a good rapport with their patient.

A lightweight mechanical massager can be gently used over the chest wall and back.

Acupressure or self-acupressure on breathless or stress points can be activated by a qualified acupuncturist or by looking at educational videos on the internet. These are;

- ➢ Cv. 17 (over the sternum at mid -nipple level)
- ➢ Lu. 1 (just below each coracoid process – which are found on the outside edge on the upper front part of the scapula/ shoulder blade)
- ➢ Bl. 13 (on each side of thoracic 3/ 4)
- ➢ Co. 4 (mid – dorsal thumb web)
- ➢ Li. 3 (on the dorsal foot between $1^{st}/ 2^{nd}$ metatarsals; proximal end).

The subject of breathlessness is also covered further in chapter six.

The Buteyko Breathing Technique

This Technique is a programme of breathing retraining which was formulated by Professor Konstantin Pavlovich Buteyko, a Ukrainian doctor, during the 1950s.

The Technique is a series of breathing exercises learnt to control rate (the speed) and volume (the size) of each breath. The breathing exercises are supplemented by other simple exercises. The exercises are specific and to be most effective need to be practised carefully and frequently over time until they become automatic.

The Technique has been most widely used by people with asthma but it has also been used by sufferers from other lung conditions, over- breathing and panic attacks. Symptoms which are addressed include wheezing, coughing, breathlessness and blocked nose. It could be that achieving good results by using the Technique's exercises could be a viable alternative, or supplement, to using bronchodilators (inhalers) and steroid medication. Obviously, before changing any medication the matter should be fully discussed with a GP and/ or consultant.

Professor Buteyko propounded from his respiratory research that over- breathing causes the production of more mucus, the constriction of bronchial tubes and the lessening of the oxygenation of the body's tissues which leads to a feeling of tiredness and feeling 'under the weather'. These three factors are especially relevant to asthma suffers in particular but they can be experienced by sufferers of other respiratory conditions.

The exercises which Buteyko devised are designed to correct an asthmatic's dysfunctional breathing pattern and help them to regain good respiratory health. Although they won't lose their allergies, the Technique's exercises will allow a sufferer's body to be better able to deal with stressful allergens and so be less likely to be triggered into an asthmatic response.

As mentioned earlier in this chapter, the Buteyko 'Control Pause Breathing Test' (CPBT) is a useful way of indicating the depth of your breathing, consequent retention of carbon dioxide, resultant oxygenation and health.

I am pleased to repeat here that my breathing capability has improved due to the work and practice I have done on my own breathing exercises. My CPBT level has improved from a 'health problems' level to a 'satisfactory health' level.

Details about the CPBT itself can be found on the website www.buteyko.co.uk.

Details of trained Buteyko teachers (including some physiotherapists) and Buteyko centres can be obtained through the Buteyko Breathing Association (www.buteykobreathing.org).

Pilates

Pilates is a unique exercise system which was devised and introduced by Joseph Pilates whose interest in breathing was influenced by his own asthmatic condition. Interestingly, the six foundations upon which Pilates is based were concepts distilled from his work by later instructors of the system.

The six Pilates Principles which are an integrative Mind, Body and Spirit holistic approach are: Centering, Concentration, Control, Precision, Breath and Flow. The Pilates exercise system which was originally called 'Contrology' by its founder can be done on exercise mats or on specially designed Pilates equipment.

While each of the six Principles are linked to each other and flow together to form a whole, the Breathing Principle emphasised a very full/ deep breath while doing exercise. Joseph Pilates advocated thinking of the lungs as a pair of bellows – using them strongly to pump the air fully into and out of the body. Most Pilates exercises co-ordinate with the breath and using the breath properly is an integral part of Pilates exercises.

Deep breathing is not just a big inhale but also a conscious effort to exhale fully which results in getting rid of every bit of stale air to allow fresh invigorating air to rush in. Joseph Pilates was adamant about the value of deep breathing. Indeed, he wrote in his book *'Return to Life Through Contrology'* that 'lazy breathing converts the lungs literally and figuratively speaking, into a cemetery for the deposition of diseased, dying and dead germs as well as supply an ideal haven for the multiplication of other harmful germs'.

When doing Pilates, and any other exercise, it is necessary to have oxygen and to get rid of carbon dioxide which is a waste product. By doing deep breathing, internal organs including the lungs and heart are stimulated and increased blood circulation will carry oxygen and nutrients to every cell with the better removal of waste products including carbon dioxide. Deep breathing is therefore the easiest and most available internal cleansing mechanism.

The Pilates system, including deep breathing, also has a body and mind integrating purpose. Joseph Pilates wanted his system to have a 'complete coordination of mind, body and spirit'. The idea that breathing fully with attention and intention is that it 'centers' us and clarifies and calms the mind. It reduces stress and leads to a greater holistic experience. Working with the breath brings a natural rhythm to bodily movement that greatly enhances a workout's efficacy and experience.

In Pilates, the breath leads movement and gives it power. To enable people to use all the available space in the lungs rather than the oft- normal upper chest there are two types of slightly different exercise which help this to be achieved. These are;

- ✓ diaphragmatic breathing – deep stomach breathing when the breath is all the way into the body, with the belly expanded with the inhale and deflated with the exhale
- ✓ lateral breathing – this is where the ribcage is expanded to allow a full intake of air.

The Alexander Technique

The Alexander Technique, which was devised and developed by Frederick Matthias Alexander, is an educational process that was created to retrain incorrect habitual patterns of movement and posture. As one of its results, it addresses many of the problems caused by an inefficient breathing pattern. The way we breathe is affected by everything we do, feel and think and vice versa.

When we make a physical effort or concentrate hard, we tend to hold our breath. Negative feelings and experiences also lead to inefficient breathing (think of the saying 'the crowd stood there with bated breath as the forward took the penalty'). If this happens a lot of times it becomes a habit and this may be done unconsciously.

Alexander deduced that poor breathing was often accompanied by a general stiffness and tension throughout the body and this can be experienced with problems such as headaches and stress.

The Alexander technique can help someone;

- ❖ understand how they can beneficially interfere with their existing inefficient breathing
- ❖ restore their natural breathing pattern
- ❖ allow the easy movement of the ribcage
- ❖ manage a number of breathing problems
- ❖ improve breathing when exercising, speaking, singing and playing wind and brass instruments.

Good breathing is a sign of equilibrium and of good physical, mental and emotional health. Sound breathing naturally supplies the amount of oxygen the body needs according to its activity at any time. Conversely, bad breathing is a sign of weakness and bad health.

Yoga

Yoga is a group of physical, mental and spiritual practices or disciplines which originated in India. Many 'modern' yoga disciplines/ styles are based on the more traditional disciplines. Some of the most popular yoga disciplines are Hatha, Vinyasa, Iyengar, Ashtanga and Bikram. Modern forms of yoga which are growing in popularity include Hot Yoga and Jojoba Chakra Yoga (details, contact www.jojobayoga.com).

Hatha Yoga, like other disciplines, stresses proper breathing and proper posture. This ancient system includes the practice of Asanas (the physical yoga postures) and Pranayama (breathing exercises).

All yoga asanas link to one or more of the body's natural energetic centres and yoga poses, breathwork and meditation techniques work to clear blockages that have developed and also release stuck energy before illness occurs. So, it follows that regular yoga practice will be associated with illness prevention.

Proper breathing and the use of correct breathing techniques during a posture is the mainstay of yoga. Hatha texts state that proper breathing exercises cleanses and balances the body. The word Pranayama is derived from 'Prana' (breath/ vital energy/ life force) & Ayama (extending and stretching).

A noted Hindu spiritual teacher and advocate of yoga Swami Sivananda said that "a yogi (a practitioner of yoga) measured the span of life by the number of breaths not by the number of years". "Perhaps if you take 15 breaths each minute you will live to 75 or 80 years of age, but if this is reduced to 10 breaths each minute you will live to 100 years of age. So, the speed of breathing will dictate the length of life; the faster you breathe the shorter the life".

Breathing consciously in yoga allows a connection with one's subtle inner energy and it is through the breath that one is able to navigate different levels of consciousness. This is in addition to the biological effect on our mental, emotional and physical health.

In a typical yoga session, students are instructed to consciously breathe, control the breath, connect to the breath, breathe deeply and retain the breath as well as doing stretching, practising postures and doing exercise.

As we saw in chapter one, conscious breathing activates a different part of the brain (the cerebral cortex and the connected areas) which is more evolved than the medulla oblongata in the brain stem which is a more primitive area of the brain. This activation relaxes and balances the emotions.

By controlling the breathing pattern, it is said that different states of mind can be achieved. Slowing breathing activates the cerebral cortex and this then sends inhibiting impulses to the respiratory centre in the midbrain. These impulses also affect and relax the hypothalamus which is concerned with emotions – therefore the emotions are relaxed with the slowing of breathing.

In yoga, the breath is the mode of Pranayama and focus is on the three stages of respiration – inhalation, retention and exhalation. Inhalation and exhalation are methods which affect retention.

Retention of breath has a physiological effect on the brain;

❖ there is more opportunity for cells to absorb oxygen and eliminate more carbon dioxide; this has a calming effect on the mental and emotional body
❖ the brain panics because the carbon dioxide level increases. This increased level stimulates the brain's capillaries to dilate and this dilation improves cerebral circulation. This leads to a large

build-up of nervous activity in the brain both forcing the creation of new neural pathways and the activation of dormant areas; the brain is awakened and the carbon dioxide level is then lowered.

Yoga can encourage breathing re-education to bring about the reduction of energy expended during breathing and also the development of relaxed breathing. The development of relaxed breathing will lead it to become deeper and slower. This will have the benefits of reducing waste energy because it doesn't need to ventilate dead space, and avoids turbulence in air flow.

The Holographic Breathing Method

This method was devised by Martin Jones about twenty years ago when he was suffering from a serious facial condition. He realised that the anatomy of the maxilla was mirrored in the appearance of the chest and lungs. He thought that the lungs were a general energy for the whole body and the sinuses were a higher energy for the brain.

Like most other systems it emphasises the importance of a relaxed body. Unlike many others there was a spiritual and emotional aspect of the breathing method. There is a great importance placed on the position of the tongue during practice and the additional important action of moving the jaw.

The connection of the person and the energy work which is a result of Martin's Method can lead to a great emotional release and connection to the mother earth, as well as being a positive physical result. Details about the Method can be found via the website: www.holographic-breathing.com.

The Objectives of this chapter were;

1. **to see in detail, how I try to improve my breathing to primarily help reduce the effects of my bronchiectasis**
2. **to understand how, with improved breathing, the respiratory system is strengthened and how this has beneficial effects on the body's general physical, mental, spiritual & emotional conditions**
3. **to give an introduction to several of the different specific breathing techniques which are available and also to several methods which emphasise the importance of breathing in their philosophy or ethos.**

CHAPTER 6: GOOD LIFESTYLE CAN HELP BRONCHIECTASIS

The Aims of the Chapter are;

1. To give an outline of how my lifestyle incorporating exercise, diet and mental positivity has helped my bronchiectasis
2. To give a description, and the benefits of different types of exercise which can be done by, and the advantages of a good lifestyle including diet and positivity for, adult & children bronchiectasis sufferers.

Introduction

Although I have been a bronchiectasis sufferer for about forty- five years, it was only diagnosed and treated in recent years. I have always exercised and kept active and have also tried to have a good diet. Added to this, I have also tried to adopt a positive attitude towards life. I feel that my approach to these three factors, which form an overall lifestyle 'package,' is why I have kept on top of its symptoms as well as I have.

I realise that my own lung health is not as bad as that of many others, but I hope that the information contained in this chapter especially about what I have done, will help them experiment and keep their symptoms at a bearable level and so improve their life. Perhaps, reading about my personal experiences, will give them the confidence and options to try things which will hopefully improve their bronchiectasis and enjoyment of life.

My lifestyle approach

Exercise and activity

Exercise is often thought of just in the context of doing sport, working out in the gymnasium or taking part in exercise classes. However, it is also an integral part of many other activities - general leisure such as gardening, DIY, making music and singing, doing housework, looking after the family and even when going on holiday (which should be relaxing, but many parts of which aren't!).

As well as taking exercise when participating in sport I also did normal energy expending activities such the gardening, walking my two dogs in the lovely woods near my home, doing DIY and going on holiday (when I walked and swam every day the sun shone). It is said that leopards can't change their spots but I have recently learnt learned the joys of ironing which I find very therapeutic (much to my wife's joy!).

Being retired, I don't have a job. When I was working, after a period of routine sedentary office work, I became a professional gardener and thereafter a physical therapist; both of these jobs entailed a lot of physical effort.

All through my life I have been interested in doing exercise in the form of playing sport to a good level and coaching and training others (adults and children) to do so. In the 1980s in London I ran the first rehabilitation and fitness gymnasium attached to a GP practice in the UK. My sports have been both team-orientated (hockey and rugby) and individual- centred (tennis, squash, badminton, golf and running).

Initially, I was interested in the competitive element of sport but as I got older, my outlook changed and it became less competitive and more of a health experience. An example of this is my regular use of a gymnasium where I have devised my own programme which is aimed at preserving my overall health rather than doing things such as building muscle mass. I was more interested in using fixed weight resistance and cardiovascular machines instead of free weights. My choice of not using free weights was mainly influenced by the fact that I had not received any tuition at an early stage about the correct techniques of using them.

My sessions in the gymnasium comprise;

1. static stretching of all muscle groups
2. cardiovascular exercise on either the static upright bike or the cross trainer
3. using weight resistance machines to strengthen all the body's muscle groups especially the chest (by using a pec deck machine), stomach, shoulders and the rear deltoids
4. a warm- down, which is either doing static stretching and/or relaxing in a warm water jacuzzi type whirlpool.

Wanting to know if exercise is helping me with my breathing as well as with my overall health, I found it important to keep an accurate record or diary of my efforts. In this respect, I would record if progress is being made or maintained. Other records I try to keep are weight, resting pulse, blood pressure and BMI. There are simple measurement machines available to the public which are relatively accurate, easy to use and not expensive. Alternatively, there are 'fit bit' type watches or health measurement apps which can be loaded on to a smart mobile phone or tablet device.

To take your own pulse reading all that is needed are two of your own fingers (not the thumb) placed on the appropriate point of the left wrist or on other pulse points located around the body and a stop watch or seconds timer on a smart phone or a clock with a second hand. The number of beats can be taken over 10 seconds and then multiplied by 6 to give a result for one minute.

Sometimes when I have exercised in the gymnasium or when doing a job, like gardening, around the house I have experienced breathlessness. My approach is to slow down or even rest for a short time and then usually recommence. By doing this, I find that I get a 'second wind' and I can complete my gym session or household job.

One of my main actions when doing any sporting exercise, whether competitively or non -competitively is to incorporate static stretching for the whole body into my routine or activity. I feel that with naturally reduced flexibility due to the ageing process this is so important. I am probably old fashioned but I feel it important to stretch both before and after doing any exercise. Looking at examples from the animal world, bats warm up before flying at night and most pet dogs stretch out first thing in the morning before becoming active. In yoga there are poses called the 'upward facing dog' (the aims of which include the improvement of breathing) and the 'downward facing dog'!

Although I had never swum competitively, now in later life I enjoy the leisure aspect of swimming and never feel intimidated or jealous of little old ladies (or men) who leave me floundering in their wake when they were doing fifty or hundred lengths of my club pool – I simply marvel at their prowess. I enjoy using a sauna (with a few drops of essential oils like eucalyptus or olbas mixed with water and added to the hot coals to then be inhaled to help clear my airways).

As well as having been a member of an excellent sports and health club at Rowton, near Shrewsbury I have assembled a number of pieces of equipment at home. These include a mini trampoline with support bar, light hand dumb bells, ergometer exercise bicycle, stomach exercisers, a Vibraplate electronic exerciser and most interesting a machine called a 'Leg Master' whose action can help to strengthen the pelvic floor and leg muscles.

While I have kitted out my own home gymnasium at a reasonable cost many of my exercises can be done by using household items such as food tins or broomsticks! Many adverts for low cost second hand fitness equipment can be found in the adverts section of local free newspapers or on eBay through the internet. Indeed, I have myself bought some excellent fitness equipment cheaply through local newspaper adverts.

There is a great amount of fitness training content available on YouTube or Instagram. In the UK, there are other free apps such as 'Couch to 5K' or Virgin's free Marathon training plan. Some companies such as 'Peloton' and individual fitness trainers like the excellent 'Mr Motivator' have beamed their lessons into people's homes via the internet during the COVID- 19 lockdown in the UK.

Inspiratory muscle exercises

I explained in chapter five how I devised a breathing pattern (Breathing Cycle Ratio Method) which best suits me and which evolved after considering a number of different methods which are available and which too are also described in brief.

As well as the general breathing exercises, I use a simple to use, hand held, small respiratory muscles training machine which is designed to make them work harder and so become stronger and more durable. The use of this trainer when combined with my use of inhaled asafoetida essential oil and the consumption of pulmonaria tea are all aimed at improving my breathing so reducing the effects of my bronchiectasis.

As well as practising my own breathing method, I try to ensure that I use it both during physical exercise and in my ordinary everyday tasks so that my gas exchange is done most efficiently and my body benefits to the maximum.

Being positive & mental exercises

I have realised that being positive means that I have to try to stay at least one step ahead of the symptoms and effects of my bronchiectasis.

I did this in the first instance by doing as much research about this nasty respiratory condition and the possible ways that its effects on me can be minimised. I realise that I will have this long-term condition with me forever and by taking this view I can be realistic about my situation.

I have been down the conventional medical treatment path which is mainly taking courses of antibiotics and doing the breathing exercises as recommended by specialist respiratory physiotherapists. This only seems to have short term positive results with recurring flare- ups happening a short time after finishing courses of medication.

It is by following my own regime that I seem to have secured as good a result as possible than by following conventional medical practice. Indeed, I haven't suffered from the adverse side effects (especially in my digestive tract) that antibiotics bring. In addition, I have probably reduced the risk of developing intolerance to their use.

By taking charge of my own health I have taken responsibility for it and this is a fantastic form of positivity. Because my methods seem to be working so well and I have a deal of knowledge about bronchiectasis which I can use, my stress levels have reduced and I am more relaxed and confident about my present and future health.

Being realistic about this condition I do know that if its symptoms and their effects are triggered and my own self- help efforts are not working, I will still be able to have access to medication which is available as a back-up.

Knowing that I have a chronic lung condition which, will always be with me and having received conventional medical treatments which have been limited to treating the symptoms rather than the cause and as they only offer a short-term solution it would have been easy for me to have suffered mentally.

Instead, I have tried to strengthen my resolve that this should not happen. Part of my solution is to keep busy mentally. As well as doing usual things such as crosswords and Sudoku, I take part in general knowledge quizzes, try to learn a foreign language and read a lot of books and magazines on a wide variety of subjects.

My mental strength follows through from my mental approach to exercising in its different forms, which I have combined with a positive approach to healthy living, including a good diet and not smoking.

Diet (food & fluids)

I know that a healthy, balanced and varied diet can nourish my body. It will not only help maintain my strength and fitness but it will also help me fight infections which will worsen any conditions such as my bronchiectasis. It will also help with my breathing because the right food is the right fuel to be used by my body for all its functions and activities including breathing.

I am very lucky to have a wonderful wife who not only is a fantastic cook but who has a similar approach to me about the importance of a good diet and healthy living.

Food

My diet provides a good, and balanced, source of protein, carbohydrates, fat, starch and unsaturated fats.

While I eat meat (both 'white' and 'red') and fish on most days, I also eat and enjoy meals which are vegetarian. I also try to eat organically produced food but because of the extra cost I find this quite difficult to do.

Although we only have a very small garden, I try to grow some of our own food and this includes strawberries, raspberries, redcurrants cherries, apples, plums, figs, tomatoes, avocados, peppers, lettuce and a number of fresh herbs. I do, of course, also grow my own pulmonaria so it can be turned into a herbal tea.

Because of the natural nutrients I take in with my balanced diet I find that I have no need to take any vitamins or nutritional supplements.

I am very conscious of my weight and I weigh myself on most days (at the same time, which for me is at the beginning of the day before breakfast). I look upon the scales as a silent friend and not something to be shied away from.

Having been tested and informed about my ideal, target weight I try to keep within a few pounds either side of that figure. If I become overweight, I know that my lungs will have to work harder to move oxygen around my body. If I become greatly underweight then I may become more susceptible to infections and by losing body mass this will include the muscles which help my breathing.

Fluids

Knowing the importance of drinking a reasonable amount of fluid to thin secretions in the lungs I normally consume drinks throughout the day starting with a cup of home produced pulmonaria tea at breakfast. My overall intake includes water, decaffeinated tea or coffee, homemade soup, soft drinks and sometimes wine, beer or spirits. My total amount probably amounts to the recommended (by the British Lung Foundation) daily intake of 7-8 cups of fluid.

Smoking

My lifetime tobacco intake has been limited to a total of about three or four small cigarillos at sports club prize awards evenings when I was in my 20s. I have regarded smoking as being damaging to my health, especially my lung health, as well as being extremely antisocial and a waste of money.

Unfortunately, my lung health had probably been seriously undermined in my early years by being exposed to the effects of my mother's passive smoking at home.

Later in this chapter I have listed many of the damaging health effects caused by the 4,000 chemicals and trace metals (which include cyanide, asbestos and many carcinogens) contained in tobacco smoke – what a horror list and not for the faint hearted!!

Sleeping

It is important to try to get as much sleep as possible to help the body and mind recover from the daily pressures and strains which are placed upon them.

I usually need about seven hours sleep nightly to allow me to function properly and the methods I use to help me include;

- ✓ having a comfortable bed and breathable memory foam mattress (which is changed approximately every eight years)
- ✓ using only one very flat pillow; in warm weather I often use a cooling gel pillow/ pad
- ✓ using bedding (duvet, sheets and pillowcases) with natural fibres which is suitable for the ambient temperature. The duvet has a Tog warmness rating thickness according to the weather
- ✓ trying to do some sleeping in a side position as well as being prone (face down)
- ✓ the bedroom has ventilation from outside
- ✓ the windows have blinds and 'blackout' curtains which block light from outside
- ✓ trying to maintain a regular time to go to bed
- ✓ wearing comfortable night clothes, which contain natural fibres, in bed
- ✓ no caffeine drink after 8pm
- ✓ not reading or using electrical, electronic or tech equipment, including radio, T.V., tablet, smart phone, computer (or similar) prior to going to sleep
- ✓ light from clocks or any other electrical equipment is kept to a minimum

- ✓ noise from clocks or fans (especially in hot weather) is minimised
- ✓ not eating any cheese for at least one hour before going to bed
- ✓ the last main meal is at least two hours before going to bed.

General good lifestyle advice

Having now read about my own experiences, I thought that it might be helpful for the reader to have some additional information which could help their bronchiectasis and its symptoms.

It is important that someone regularly puts into practice whatever they decide is best for them to achieve their aims, but they should still be able to incorporate flexibility into their approach. These elements are;

- physical exercise and activity
- diet
- smoking
- sleeping
- mental positivity
- possible incontinence

I have looked at the situation relating to adults and children with bronchiectasis separately as their needs are different and the approach to meeting the needs of these two age groups may have to be modified.

Adults

Physical exercise and activity

Before undertaking exercise in any of its many forms, it is important to discuss your limitations, needs, aims and aspirations with either your GP or respiratory expert as they be able to offer advice based on their skill, knowledge and experience which may be pertinent to your plans.

Exercise can have a lot of benefits and these include;

1. increasing lung volume by combining an upright posture (either standing or in a supportive chair) with an improved deep breathing process
2. strengthening muscles so that oxygen is used more efficiently, with the lungs not having to work so hard when you are being active
3. improving overall physical fitness and flexibility
4. the ability to fight infections better
5. improving confidence and a sense of wellbeing which in turn reduces anxiety and depression
6. reduces the perception of breathlessness
7. posture improves and everyday tasks such as walking and shopping should become easier and better
8. reduces the need for and 'enjoyment' of smoking; so helping relaxation, sleeping, regulation of blood sugar levels and gut problems
9. managing and coping with incontinence related to bronchiectasis

Research has shown the many specific respiratory benefits of regular exercise and these include;

- breathing capacity can be increased. With low intensity exercise, increased deeper breathing is most important; at high intensity, fast breathing is the most important
- previously closed lung capillaries are opened and muscle blood flow can increase dramatically (x25)
- oxygen take up is increased in the body by up to 20-fold
- bronchodilation occurs in healthy lungs
- better mucus transport.

For people with respiratory conditions, like bronchiectasis, aerobic (with oxygen) endurance training which comprises high – repetition, low - resistance exercise is more suitable than strength training which comprises low- repetition, high – resistance exercise because this will enhance the use of available oxygen. However, it is a good idea that some strength training be combined with endurance training to make things less boring and possibly reduce the risk of repetitive strain injuries.

Isotonic exercise (when a contracting muscle shortens against a constant load e.g. a biceps curl) rather than isometric exercise (static contraction of a muscle without any visible movement in the angle of a joint e.g. a side 'plank') is preferred as this is more vigorous. Exercise levels should be gradually built up to achieve the individual's reasonable goal levels. It should be done steadily with rest breaks being incorporated in any session and competition with others should usually not be encouraged.

As well as the exercise activity part of any exercise session there should also be a warm- up and cool-down at the beginning and end of the activity. It is important to incorporate some stretching exercises into these. Static stretching can be done before starting any activity; for example, climbing a ladder can be preceded by stretching the calf muscles as these will become under load.

It is important that water is taken in before and during the session to reduce the risk of dehydration and at any time the participant can stop doing the exercise if they feel unwell.

I have already mentioned that I exercise my respiratory muscles by using a small, inexpensive device.

Inspiratory muscle training can be helpful for people who need to be desensitized to breathlessness, who may have difficulty in changing their breathing pattern or who simply enjoy the process.

Exercise can also have many social benefits if it is done in a group or class setting or in the company of an empathetic trainer on a one to one basis.

Breathlessness

In addition, any exercise, such as walking and swimming (which has the benefit of being weight bearing) which makes someone slightly breathless is extremely good for bronchiectasis sufferers because it will help clear the chest. The level of breathlessness while exercising varies between individuals and generalisations about this sensation can be misleading.

It is advisable that the sensation of breathlessness is introduced to a sufferer in a controlled manner. By doing this, the sufferer will learn and know about his/her capacity and will recognise the signs of 'overdoing 'things and will be able to cope with potentially stressful situations better. The sufferer knows his own capabilities best and if he/ she feels they are being exceeded then a certain exercise or activity should be stopped or adjustments made.

The subject of breathlessness is also covered in detail later and in chapter five.

Introduction to exercise

There are two good alternative ways of getting formally introduced to exercise which is planned to improve the function of the pulmonary (heart and lungs) system.

Initially, a specialist respiratory physiotherapist, consultant or GP will advise on the best and most appropriate exercises for a patient. He/ she can refer a patient to a specialist Pulmonary Rehabilitation (PR) exercise group programme which usually run at a local hospital, community venue or leisure centre and usually has between 8 – 16 participants.

This formal PR programme, which is led and supervised by a qualified respiratory professional, lasts for six to eight weeks and involves both aerobic and resistance/ strength training and should include the elements of intensity, frequency, duration, type, mode and progression. The modes of aerobic training are walking (ground-based or treadmill), static cycling or rower. Strength training is designed to improve muscle strength and endurance and works muscle groups in the trunk, upper and lower limbs.

To assist respiratory function, mobilising exercises for the thoracic spine and rib cage can be learnt on the programme. These exercises can either be incorporated into the warm- up and cool- down or done separately.

The PR programme will be tailored to meet the individual's needs and incorporates a physical exercise programme designed for people living with lung conditions. Anyone suffering from breathlessness, due to different respiratory conditions, may also benefit from the formal exercise or pulmonary rehabilitation programme.

Pulmonary rehabilitation is aimed at;

- an improvement in the ability to exercise (exercise tolerance)
- an improvement in health-related quality of life

- the possibility of reducing the annual number of chest infections
- reducing the number of visits to the GP or hospital.

The physiotherapist will be able to;

✓ give advice about looking after your body and lungs
✓ explain how to manage a specific respiratory condition such as bronchiectasis
✓ advise on how to cope with feeling short of breath, including positions to help relieve breathlessness and how to pace yourself
✓ advise on breathing techniques to help control your breathing.

As well as doing group exercises, there are significant educational and social benefits of the PR Programme.

A participant is observed when exercising and there is an opportunity to ask the course leader questions such as "what level of breathlessness is good for me?" and "are there any exercises which can be done if other health problems prevent me doing the programme's exercises?".

Exercise capacity measurements could be carried out and these include a 6-minute walk test (6MWT) or the incremental shuttle walk test (ISWT).

A second option is for the sufferer to be referred by a GP (at no cost to the GP) to an approved venue (sports club, clinic, sports centre or gymnasium) to take part in a 12 week 'Fitness on Prescription' (or similar titled) programme. On this programme, a patient has a number of personalised training sessions with an accredited qualified instructor. Normally, the venue allows the patient to pay a reduced temporary membership fee during the duration of the programme.

In Australia (see www.bronchiectasis.com.au) exercise or physical activity is seen to be one of the foundations of healthy living in its population and particularly with those suffering from respiratory conditions such as bronchiectasis. They have drawn up national guidelines for physical activity and sedentary behaviour and these are a good place to see how a physical activity programme for an individual can be developed.

Diet

Food

There is a saying which is 'you are what you eat'. While in theory we should all have a diet which is balanced, varied and good for us, in practice this is often difficult to achieve and maintain. There are many factors to take into account and these include;

- level of income and disposable income for food and drink
- availability and cost of food ingredients e.g. the (usually) extra financial cost of organic food products
- availability of cooking equipment
- time available for cooking & consuming meals
- cooking skill level

- level of knowledge about food and drink and how they influence health
- cultural background, location and lifestyle e.g. ethnicity, vegetarianism and veganism
- peer and family pressures
- eating habits and times
- food allergies and intolerances
- other health issues including long- or short-term stress, mental, emotional or physical problems (e.g. type 2 diabetes) or a combination of these.

A balanced and varied diet can help achieve and maintain strength and fitness and as food is the fuel used by bodily functions including breathing the right mix can assist breathing. Whilst general advice about food and diet should be the same as for the public as a whole it should be remembered that sufferers of bronchiectasis have special needs.

Different food groups carry out different functions and these include;

- ✓ proteins which are needed for healthy muscles and should be consumed twice daily e.g. meat, fish, eggs, cheese, milk, nuts and lentils
- ✓ carbohydrates, including starchy & sugary foods which are the major source of body energy
- ✓ starchy foods could be eaten at each meal e.g. bread, potatoes, rice, pasta and cereals
- ✓ sugary foods e.g. cake and biscuits can provide additional short-term energy but must be consumed with care to prevent obesity, poor dental health and other serious health issues

- ✓ fat (preferably unsaturated fat) is a concentrated form of energy e.g. butter, margarine, vegetable oil and cream.

A healthy diet should preferably incorporate;

- ✓ fresher instead of processed food
- ✓ more whole foods
- ✓ a reduction of salt content
- ✓ fibre in the form of fruit, vegetables and whole grains.
- ✓ five portions of fruit and vegetables daily. One of the benefits of vitamin C, which is contained in many citrus fruits, is that it helps mucus transport.

Sometimes it is difficult to meet energy needs from existing foods which are being consumed. If this is the case a doctor, nutritionist or dietician may be able to offer advice on any helpful dietary changes that should be made including taking nutritional products including mineral and vitamin supplements.

Drinking fluids

By drinking fluids throughout the day this should help thin secretions in the lungs and make it easier to cough them up. This will help reduce the risk of infections. It has been recommended that a daily intake of 7-8 cups of healthy fluid should be consumed. If drinking fluid with meals causes problems then a limit should be imposed and a drink should be taken an hour after eating. The timing of when best to drink (and eat) and the benefits of different types of drink is a complicated subject and an NHS expert should be able to advise about this subject.

The question of weight

Obese and overweight people generally have lower lung volumes and reduced lung and chest wall inelasticity/ compliance and this helps makes their action inefficient so leading to rapid and shallow breathing patterns.

On the other hand, malnourished people are not able to improve muscle function and exercise tolerance without gaining weight.

Because of the importance of knowing about your weight, this should be regularly measured on scales. The best time is to do this after getting up in the morning before having breakfast (if you are a shift worker a variation of meal should be made). Look upon the scales as 'being one of your best friends'.

It is worth repeating that unexpected changes in weight could be significant to a bronchiectasis sufferer. Becoming overweight means that the heart and lungs will have to work harder to supply oxygen to all parts of the body. Becoming underweight or losing weight may lead to more risk of infections. Loss of muscle mass will weaken the muscles which help with breathing.

If you are overweight, then losing excess weight through a healthy diet and exercise will help make breathing easier. This can be done by reducing the intake of fatty and sugary foods. A reduction in both portion size and grazing between meals could also be positive dietary tools. Older people must take care because it has been suggested that grazing between meals may not be a positive thing.

Unexpected weight loss could lead to you feeling weaker. To gain weight and feel stronger, consumption of energy foods (including high fat foods) and protein could be increased. If there are breathing problems the sufferer could use more energy than a healthy person. Similarly, fighting chest infections could use up a lot of available energy.

Change in meals routine

Breathlessness may lead to eating becoming more difficult and also a loss of appetite. If this happens then someone could try eating three smaller nutrient dense meals daily with additional snacks or milky drinks (now there are substitutes to cow's milk on sale) between meals. Softer foods which require less effort in chewing may be easier to eat and digest.

There are some specific foods the reduction of intake of which a sufferer could experiment with for a length of time (say 3-4 weeks) to see if they benefit from the change in diet. These are;

- ✓ dairy foods because it has been claimed that they increase the viscosity in mucus
- ✓ caffeine in drinks
- ✓ alcohol
- ✓ spicy foods and additives (e.g. monosodium glutamate).

Smoking

It is vital that bronchiectasis sufferers cease smoking because;

- their prognosis (the likely course of a condition) is improved,
- lung irritation is avoided
- there will be less chance of developing other lung damage including COPD (Chronic Obstructive Pulmonary Disease) or lung cancer
- otherwise there will an increase in airways obstruction
- otherwise damage will be done to the alveoli's surfactant fluid (made up of lipids and proteins) which is needed to lower the work of breathing and prevents alveolar collapse at the end of expiration.

Smoking, and passive smoking, brings many other health problems including;

- increased lower back pain
- the main risk factor for postoperative chest infection
- increased infant mortality, incidence of childhood respiratory diseases and lung development

- accelerates ageing
- raises blood pressure
- causes eye cataract, squint and glue ear in many children
- dislodges teeth and ulcerates the gut
- doubles or triples female infertility and leads to a high incidence of male sperm abnormalities
- reduction in appetite, which is important for malnourished people
- ……. need any more!!

Fortunately, there are a large number of methods available to those who want to stop smoking and the first port of call should be the GP, Practice Nurse or pharmacy to seek their advice and support.

Sleeping

The importance of good sleeping cannot be exaggerated and there have been very many studies, books and internet articles to this effect. For those suffering from bronchiectasis and other respiratory conditions, the significance of trying to incorporate the side- lying position when sleeping, because of its significant physical breathing benefits it can bring, is important.

A number of suggestions about steps to help sleeping are listed earlier in the chapter (page 241).

Mental positivity

In chapter two and also earlier in this chapter, we looked at the importance of positivity and how it has been used to help me and has the potential to help other bronchiectasis sufferers.

Often people think they are alone with a problem especially a medical one such as bronchiectasis which currently has no cure and the best is that its symptoms can be mainly alleviated by medication and physiotherapy.

The main thing is to be positive and take advantage of any help or advice which is available to reduce the effects of the condition. Do not needlessly suffer alone or allow those close to you to suffer as well.

Firstly, ensure that you have exhausted all avenues of guidance, help and advice which can be offered by;

- your GP
- your respiratory consultant
- your local hospital respiratory physiotherapy department
- in some areas in the UK (e.g. Lothian, Scotland) there are teams of health-care workers (nurse, physiotherapist, respiratory doctors, GP and consultant) to help bronchiectasis patients
- charities and organisations such as the British Lung Foundation and the British Thoracic Society who specialise in respiratory conditions
- local Breathing Clubs which offer support, physical activities and social contact.

Secondly, as well as taking advantage of the benefits of the above types of organisation and specialists there are many things you can do yourself which will allow you to take responsibility for your own health such as;

- ✓ monitoring your own health by using equipment which is available
- ✓ eating and drinking as well as circumstances and finances allow
- ✓ stopping smoking and avoiding situations which may worsen the bronchiectasis
- ✓ doing appropriate exercise which could range from doing simply walking more or joining a sports club which offers a variety of exercise facilities
- ✓ trying to do mental puzzles and problems such as jigsaws and crosswords which exercise the brain or take up a hobby such as painting, chess, music or cooking which broadens the mind and increases the skill set. Joining a hobby club(s) offers a new dimension to the mind and is a social activity
- ✓ volunteering your time in a responsible way which offers the opportunity for a reasonable level of exercise and exertion as well as the chance to meet other people
- ✓ joining patient support groups either locally or online through which you may get reassurance about any worries you may have and also have the opportunity of learning and sharing experiences about the condition.

Incontinence linked to bronchiectasis

Many women and men of all ages and with different medical conditions, including bronchiectasis, asthma and COPD, suffer with a constant, chronic cough and related Urinary incontinence (Ui) which is an embarrassing leakage of urine. Please also see page 51.

Ui has a wide spectrum of severity and nature and in less serious cases there can be a number of self- help measures that can be taken including doing bladder muscle (Kegel) exercises, losing weight, eating more fibre and avoiding certain foods.

This is a common problem which is difficult to cope with in everyday life; in the case of those with bronchiectasis It may lead to a reluctance to do necessary airway clearance.

For bronchiectasis sufferers in particular, and those with more serious symptoms, if incontinence happens it is important to ask for help. Advice from a physiotherapist or continence nurse who specialises in this field should help.

There are also available different types of health products which could be tried. The 'Innovo' is a clinically proven device to restore the pelvic floor muscles so treating the cause of urinary leaks. Another machine is the 'Leg Master' which works this area while it is being used during exercise.

Children

In Australia, the philosophy of encouraging physical activity and looking at sedentary behaviour is also followed to help children with mild bronchiectasis. Hopefully, they will only have a minimal limitation on activity and vigorous sports and games can be adapted to meet their needs. Their exercise prescription will depend on age and clinical status and should include elements of cardiovascular & endurance training, muscle training and mobility exercises.

Toddlers and young children have fun physical activities incorporated into their physiotherapy treatment time. Changes in airflow and volume and mucus clearance can be aimed at for example when they are bouncing on a large therapy 'Swiss' ball. Soccer and chase tag games as well as chest percussion are all aimed at helping mucus clearance.

Fun and age-appropriate activities such as 'wheelbarrows', 'mimicked boxing' and safe easy wall climbing incorporate upper body strengthening and stretching.

Children's exercise can be seen as the basis of airway clearance therapy and can be combined with other techniques. When done in different positions the effects of gravity come into play. Exercise can be done either before or after airway clearance techniques. If possible, physical exercise or thoracic expansion exercises should be done at the end of a session so leaving the airways as open as possible.

Physical exercise for children has a number of benefits and these include;

- it is a stimulating airway clearance alternative involving parents, siblings and friends
- it is a time- efficient airway clearance therapy
- different exercises can be easily replaced to give variety or when needed
- varied exercise will help children stay interested in their treatment
- expensive equipment or a large space is not necessary
- quality of life and general wellbeing is improved
- weight- bearing exercise increases bone mineral density which has long term benefit
- friends are made at a creche, preschool or school – this benefit can accrue to parents and carers as well.

Useful hints

- children should be encouraged to exercise several times weekly
- it is important they drink adequate water before, during and after exercise
- stretching is important
- some children may need to use bronchodilators before exercise
- family members and friends should be included in any exercise sessions.

Part of the excellent Lung Foundation of Australia website: (www.lungfoundation.com.au/research/our-research/bronchiectasis) is a section about children's (paediatric) bronchiectasis. You access the Bronchiectasis Toolbox section of the website and you will find three relevant sections full of useful example about children;

- assessment and management
- exercises
- action plan & care plan.

The Aims of the Chapter were;

1. **To give an outline of how my own overall lifestyle, which incorporates exercise and activity, diet and mental positivity, has helped my own bronchiectasis and its symptoms**
2. **To give general information and advice about how exercise, diet and positivity can help adult and children bronchiectasis sufferers.**

CHAPTER 7: POST NASAL DRIP AND BRONCHIECTASIS

The Aims of this Chapter are;

1. **to describe how I tried to improve my bronchiectasis by reducing my post nasal drip condition**
2. **to explain what post nasal drip is and how its actions can have an effect on bronchiectasis**
3. **to give a brief introduction to some of the methods which can be tried to reduce the incidence of post nasal drip.**

Introduction

Post Nasal Drip (PND) which is also known as Upper Airway Cough Syndrome (UACS) or Post Nasal Drip Syndrome (PNDS) happens when excessive mucus secretions are produced by the nasal and paranasal sinuses mucosa. These mucosae are linings of the cavities and are made up of ciliated epithelium with goblet cells and they warm and humidify inhaled air and sweep dust and microbes to the pharynx.

The secretions stimulate the upper airway cough receptors and the resulting inflammation increases receptor sensitivity. The mucus produced in the sinuses (which drain into the back of the nose) and nasal area accumulates in the back of the nose and then moves into the throat after being dripped down.

Mucus is a thick, semi -fluid wet slimy discharge from the nose that moistens the throat and airways as well as the nose itself. It helps to trap and destroy foreign bodies such as bacteria, viruses and other foreign matter before they cause infection.

Mucus from the nose usually mixes with saliva, drips harmlessly down the back of the throat and is then swallowed. More or thicker mucus than normal becomes noticeable. Excess which comes out of the nostrils is called a 'runny' nose. When excess mucus runs down the back of the nose to the throat it is called postnasal drip.

There are a lot of causes for Post Nasal Drip (PND) and these include;

- rhinitis (inflammation of the mucous membrane which lines the nose)
- sinusitis (inflammation of the membrane lining the facial sinuses)
- a deviated septum, with one nasal passage smaller than the other
- gastroesophageal reflux disease (GERD) and other swallowing disorders such as gastric acid reflux (which causes throat irritation leading to the sensation of increased mucus in the throat
- allergies (including a reaction to birth control pills (which can be switched by a GP, or by using an alternative form of birth control). This could be called allergic PND
- viral infections leading to colds and flu
- hormonal changes experienced during pregnancy, menopause or menstruation
- side effects from medications including some birth control and blood pressure prescriptions

- dry air in the home or in the workplace
- cold temperatures and changes in the weather (especially in the spring & summer)
- a reaction to spicy foods which may trigger mucus flow
- fumes from chemicals, cleaning products, strong perfume, smoke or other irritants
- objects stuck up the nose, which is more common in children.

Sometimes the problem causing PND isn't the excessive mucus, but the throat's inability to clear it. Swallowing problems or gastric reflux can cause liquid to build up in the throat which can feel like PND.

How I tried to reduce my Post Nasal Drip

Early in this book's foreword you may recall that I wrote that a specialist respiratory doctor used the term 'Post Nasal Drip' when talking about me while I was being treated for breathing problems when I was a teenager at secondary school.

I have many of the classic symptoms of PND which I feel are linked with, and exacerbate, my bronchiectasis. These symptoms are;

- sore throat
- coughing, especially through the night
- a feeling of general discomfort in both the upper airways and the lungs which includes a feeling of the whole system being overwhelmed by a fullness of fluid, akin to being drowned

- 'tickle' in the throat
- constant throat clearing or swallowing
- congestion in the upper airways - nasal and/or paranasal sinus passages,
- a 'metallic' mucus feeling in the back of the throat.

I unsuccessfully had different medical treatments for PND – decongestants, antihistamines and minor surgery as well as using a 'Neti pot' nasal wash at home. I thought thereafter that I would take a different approach to try to interrupt the downward flow of mucus from the nasal and sinuses passages into the throat which takes place while I am awake and also while I am asleep.

I also decided to try to change my lifestyle so that my symptoms would not get worse.

Looking at the composition of the mucus which was produced and removed from the nasal passage and that which was produced in my lungs they seemed to be very similar in consistency and colour and this suggested that there could be a strong link between the two areas.

I wondered how I could reduce the amount of mucus flowing down into my throat and the solutions I came up with were simple and these were;

- ✓ using the asafoedita essential oil vapour inhalation. As well as drawing out fluid from the lungs and lower airways, there was an additional beneficial effect on the state of the nasal and sinuses passages because mucus which had been loosened during the inhalations was removed by blowing my nose. This mucus was either clear or with an infection colour and thicker consistency

✓ removal of nasal/ sinus mucus could be triggered by the simple action of rolling the edge of a tissue into a point and inserting it in turn up each nostril. After doing this stimulation for a short time, mucus (clear or otherwise) would start to flow and could be removed by the action of blowing the nose with the tissue (which is then hygienically disposed of). Often this flowing action is preceded by a loud sneeze!

By doing both of the above actions, mucus in the sinuses and nasal areas would be removed and lessened and would not be available to flow down the throat while being either asleep or awake.

It is often recommended that people could try propping up their pillows at night so that mucus won't pool or collect in the back of the throat. I take a contrary view; in bed I sleep as flat as possible (on one very thin pillow). Not only does this seem to be a better neutral angle for the neck thus causing less strain on it but gravity is not able to help mucus fluid flow down towards the throat and thereafter some to the stomach and the rest down towards the airways and lungs.

Obviously, many people will not be able to sleep (almost) flat for medical reasons. Perhaps for them a reduction from two (or three) pillows down to one could be tried for a couple of weeks to see if any beneficial change occurs – if nothing positive happens, the sleeper can revert back to two (or three) pillows.

Having reached the age of 71 I found, like many other men (and women) of this age and sometimes younger/ older that I have to visit the bathroom during the night. Whilst one of the things I have to do during my nocturnal perambulation is to empty my bladder by peeing out my urine I have often experienced the need to either cough out phlegm or blow my nose to clear my nasal and sinus airways.

It would probably be useful to learn which of these three actions the brain thinks is the most vital. I would think that it perceives the improvement of the respiratory system taking precedence over the working of the urinary system.

Fluid intake

One of the best kitchen appliances we have is a cheap soup making machine. This machine very quickly turns a range of vegetable and cooked meat/ fish ingredients into a meal which is not only nutritious, tasty and cheap but because it is a hot liquid its heat opens up my stuffy nose and also helps prevent dehydration. These health (and financial) benefits should help make you (and your finances) feel better. If anyone is following either a vegetarian or vegan diet then the soup's ingredients can be modified accordingly to suit their diet.

I also tried to vary my diet by reducing the intake of dairy products especially milk. The drinking of pulmonaria tea (with no added milk) was one way of doing this.

General information about Post Nasal Drip (PND)

Symptoms of Post Nasal Drip

The symptoms of Post Nasal Drip include;

- hoarseness and a sore throat
- coughing (which is the result of the transportation of mucus from the nasal membranes down the back of the throat so triggering a cough) can lead to soreness
- constant congestion and throat clearing
- constant difficulty in swallowing and a dry mouth
- nasal & paranasal sinuses passage congestion
- a runny nose
- sneezing
- a feeling of mucus in the throat
- the sensation of a lump in the back of the throat
- nausea caused by some of the excess mucus moving into the stomach
- fatigue, mainly due to interruptions to a sleep pattern, caused by the condition
- face pain or pressure or fullness
- severe bad breath (halitosis).
- change in smell (hyposmia- which is a reduced ability to smell and detect odours).

Any of these symptoms can be increased during an allergy season.

Methods to try to reduce Post Nasal Drip

There are a number of different methods which can be tried to reduce Post Nasal Drip and its effects. These methods can be categorised into;

- conventional medical treatments
- complementary and alternative treatments
- lifestyle changes.

Conventional medical treatments

Medication

Certain decongestants, such as Pseudoephedrine (Sudafed), are prescribed to treat PND. This decongestant drug is aimed at relieving the stuffy and runny nose symptoms by causing a reduction in the membranes through the tightening of blood vessels in a membrane.

Non- drowsy antihistamines such as loratadine-pseudoephedrine (Claritin) helps to get rid of PND and these become more effective after they are taken for several days. Antihistamines are also recommended if the PND is caused by allergies.

GPs often prescribe cortisone steroid nasal sprays. These sprays are safe and more effective than over-the- counter decongestant sprays which can be bought in a pharmacy and which have a more limited time of being helpful.

If the PND is the result of a bacterial infection or is linked to sinusitis, antibiotics can be prescribed.

If the feeling of PND could be caused by other conditions such as acid reflux, GERD (gastroesophageal reflux disease) or trouble with swallowing, a GP can organise tests and prescribe appropriate medication.

Surgery

Minor surgery can be done to open blocked sinuses and to help their drainage. If PND is caused by a deviated septum, corrective surgery may be the only way to permanently treat it. This surgery (a septoplasty) tightens and straightens the nasal septum. This procedure may involve the removal of parts of the septum.

There are several types of sinus irrigation surgery and this is only done after other treatments have been tried. The sinus cavities are rinsed to flush out all the infected and excess mucus. Your GP will advise on the most appropriate and on the after- care which has to be done by the patient.

Complementary and alternative treatments

An ancient treatment is the use of a 'Neti Pot' which is filled with a saline solution to rinse the nasal passages so helping the drainage of thick mucus which has become stuck. The 'Neilmed sinus rinse' is a system whereby a saline solution irrigates the nasal passage and excretes or removes the accumulation of the mucus in the area. This system is recommended by many GPs and is available at pharmacies and other similar outlets.

To alleviate bad breath due to PND you can try rinsing with a warm salt water gargle. Alternatively, there are refreshing throat sprays available.

Many complementary therapies such as reflexology, acupressure and acupuncture are used to treat nasal and sinus complaints as well as other respiratory conditions. Other practitioners such as osteopaths, chiropractors, herbalists, homeopaths and Traditional Chinese Medicine (TCM) can also be consulted as their expertise includes (often specialised) treatments of respiratory conditions.

Lifestyle changes

A good way to prevent PND is to reduce exposure to allergens as much as possible, this can be done in many ways including;

- ✓ keep your home and workplace as clean and dust free as possible and use a vacuum cleaner which

gives good results collecting pet's moulted fur and hairs
- ✓ take a daily allergy medication and get any regular allergy injections; sometimes better results will be achieved before any known allergy season begins
- ✓ use mattress and pillow covers to protect against dust mites and keep all bedding as clean as possible
- ✓ shower before going to bed if you have spent a long time outside especially if you are allergic to dust, pollen, spores or feathers/fur
- ✓ air filters on heating, ventilation and air conditioning units should be cleaned or changed regularly
- ✓ use breathing protection with clean filters if you are working in a dusty environment at work or when doing gardening, DIY and hobbies at home such as woodworking.

Staying hydrated can help both prevent and treat PND. Drinking warm or hot liquid such as tea or chicken soup can thin out mucus and prevents dehydration. Drinking sufficient water also thins out mucus and keeps the throat moistened. Alcohol and caffeine-based drinks can worsen symptoms so should be minimised.

The Aims of this Chapter were;

1. to describe how I tried to reduce the effects on my bronchiectasis of my bronchiectasis by lessening my post nasal drip

2. to explain what post nasal drip is and how its actions can have an effect on bronchiectasis
3. to give a brief introduction to some of the different methods which can try to reduce the incidence of post nasal drip.

CONCLUSION

Well, here we are at the end of the book about my journey to try and find a method or programme to combat my bronchiectasis and the long-term effects it has wrought not only on my own health and life but also on the life of my family.

I realised that this respiratory condition was long term foe and while I (or anybody else) couldn't cure it, by following my own programme I was confident that I could improve my situation. Having achieved this with a lot of effort and changes in my lifestyle I think that I have truly 'TAMED IT' as I set out so to do.

I realise that bronchiectasis, like other respiratory conditions, affects sufferers in different ways and to different degrees. I hope that you will find details of what I did helpful to you and if you try some of things I did, this may help your health progress through life. Some of my actions such as using asafoedita oil vapour inhalation and drinking pulmonaria tea are quite radical and probably ground- breaking but as they worked for me, they may be the things you have been missing to **improve your life**.

I thought it right to look at bronchiectasis in the whole, and to this end I have given the reader a lot of background information about the condition – what it is; what causes it; its symptoms; other treatments for it and research into it. Many interesting items are raised including: the importance of the body's natural nitric oxide; the good clearance of sputum due to exercise and correct, deep breathing; the long- term bad effects of passive smoking on the respiratory health of all, especially babies, toddlers and young people; the suppression of the immune system by the presence of the PZP protein.

Many treatments that are written up often rely on anecdotal comments or are based on an insufficient data base. In my case all I can say and stress is;

1. I hadn't taken any medication (including antibiotics) for my bronchiectasis for a period of about 5 years. When I recently did take some, they had adverse side effects
2. a spirometry test carried out on me recently before a major operation at my local orthopaedic hospital gave a reading that my lung age was 10 years below my actual age; furthermore, the nurse conducting the test said that my result was positivity almost off the scale!
3. the use of my programme was probably a contributory factor in getting another objective test measurement which placed my metabolic age at 15 years less than my birth age!!
4. I breathe more easily in stressful situations, such as when I have to sit still for quite a while when my mouth is being irrigated and full of water during a dental treatment
5. While my programme has involved hard work and patience; its good results have improved my mental attitude towards the condition and its symptoms and I do not have to be solely reliant on medical intervention (although it is available as a possible backup).

Good luck with your own future bronchiectasis health.

APPENDIX

BRONCHIECTASIS RESEARCH

Introduction

Details of some UK and worldwide general research into bronchiectasis is contained in this Appendix. Although details about this research may appear dry and can be skipped over by the reader, it could prove to be interesting to any bronchiectasis sufferer (and hopefully some respiratory practitioners).

Many bronchiectasis sufferers have had a feeling of being alone with their condition and that compared with sufferers of other more publicised health conditions and diseases they, and their condition, have not counted for much. A simple example of this can be seen in the fact that generally most people have heard of bronchitis, asthma or COPD but how many have heard of bronchiectasis?

Hopefully, the details about the wide-ranging bronchiectasis research which has been carried out internationally, some of which is described below, will give sufferers hope that things will improve for them, as well as enabling the condition to become better known, understood and planned for and treated. It is also important to mention two of the pioneers of bronchiectasis research.

Ground breaking bronchiectasis researchers

Historically, two of the most ground breaking researchers into the condition were **René - Théophile-Hyacinthe Laennec (1781 – 1826)** and **Sir William Osler (1849 -1919)**. Laennec was a French physician, musician and philanthropist who invented the stethoscope in 1816 and used his invention to first diagnose bronchiectasis in 1819. He died of tuberculosis. Osler, an eminent Canadian physician, writer and teacher and a founding father of the John Hopkins Hospital, Baltimore researched bronchiectasis in great detail in the late 1800s. He suffered with continual chest infections and died during the Spanish flu pandemic from suspected undiagnosed bronchiectasis. Having looked at the internet and viewed YouTube content about these two fascinating individuals I would recommend any reader to look them up – time will be well spent in so doing.

Worldwide general bronchiectasis studies including the underestimation of its prevalence, incidence and mortality

Up until recent times there has been a culture of underestimating the significance of bronchiectasis in its prevalence (number of cases), incidence (number of newly diagnosed cases), mortality and analysis of those affected. This has been important, because in the past it has been considered as an 'orphan' condition with a relatively small number of sufferers.

There have been a number of recent reports, papers and articles about bronchiectasis, produced in diverse countries such as the UK, the USA, Australia, New Zealand, Germany, South Korea and Catalonia (Spain) and the statistics and findings in many of these dispute some of the existing assumptions about the condition.

By accepting previous thinking on this matter, many governments and their health departments have not implemented appropriate policies and forward planning to cater for the actual greater number, and types, of sufferers than previously thought.

Often there are common generalised trends in the reports' findings and these are described, after examples of the individual reports are outlined and how they can be accessed.

In the United Kingdom there a number of national and local charities and other medical organisations and self-help groups who give advice, carry out research or disseminate information about chronic respiratory conditions including bronchiectasis. These charities include the British Lung Foundation (www.blf.org.uk) and their advice can be accessed through the internet, by telephone or by reading their helpful printed leaflets.

The Foundation sponsored a study *'Epidemiology of bronchiectasis in the UK: Findings from the British Lung Foundation's 'Respiratory Health of the Nation'* project by teams at George's Hospital University of London, Nottingham University and Imperial College

London. The data, covering the years between 2004 and 2012, and the study's findings were published in the journal *Respiratory Medicine*. The following were found;

- in 2012, approximately 210,000 people were living with bronchiectasis which was at least four times higher than the NHS estimate of approximately 50,000
- in 2004, 230 per 100,000 were diagnosed; in 2010, 303 per 100,000; 2012, 320 per 100,000
- between 2008 and 2012 prevalence increased by 20% (40,000)
- the highest proportion affected was in the West Midlands; the lowest was in the South East
- the rate for first diagnosis of bronchiectasis in primary care increased from 20 to 33 people per 100,000 between 2004 and 2012
- in 2012 there were 20% more women than men diagnosed for the first time with bronchiectasis. Every year there are always more cases diagnosed among females than males; around 35% more women than men are diagnosed each year
- around 60% of bronchiectasis diagnoses are made in people aged over 70, diagnosis is more likely as you get older between ages of 30 and 70
- the number of people who died from bronchiectasis increased from 1,150 in 2008 to 1,567 in 2012. Of these deaths 123 were 15-64 years and the remainder were aged 65 and older

- the regions with lower death rates from bronchiectasis than the UK average were the East of England, London and the South West.

A paper *'Changes in the incidence, prevalence and mortality of bronchiectasis in the UK from 2004 to 2013: a population- based cohort study'* by Quint J.K. et al (based on CPRD: Clinical Practice Research Datalink) was published in the European Respiratory Society's [(ERS), Email: journals@ersnet.org] *European Respiratory Journal 2016 47: 186-193* and it suggested that numbers having bronchiectasis in the UK could have increased to approximately 300,000.

This paper states that there is a paucity of data about incidence, prevalence and mortality associated with non-cystic fibrosis (CF) bronchiectasis. This report also admits that there are major deficits in the understanding and management of the condition. As bronchiectasis remains an important cause of respiratory disease in the UK this should be reflected in the provision of clinical care for sufferers.

The increase in bronchiectasis incidence and prevalence could be for several reasons including the reclassification of respiratory diseases, a better understanding and diagnosis of the condition and older adult-onset.

However, it determined;

✓ the total number of people living with bronchiectasis in the UK in 2013 was estimated to

be 300,000 (rounded down to the nearest 100,000) comprising 485.5 males per 100,000 males = 153,107; and 566.1 females per 100,000 females = 184,377. This totals 337,484 which exceeds the previous estimate for 2012 of 210,00 as shown above in the British Lung Foundation sponsored research
- ✓ there was an annual increase yearly in the study period across all age groups and in both sexes
- ✓ bronchiectasis is common and increasing, particularly in older age groups
- ✓ in all age bands, mortality rates were substantially higher (more than twice) when compared with the general population
- ✓ an increase in bronchiectasis in almost all age groups with the most rapid increase in women over 70 years
- ✓ a diagnosis has important health implications especially on mortality rates
- ✓ as there are more CT scans performed in the HIV population, this probably accounts for the higher rate in this group
- ✓ bronchiectasis is deemed to be idiopathic (the cause is unknown) if it is not associated with any of the common comorbidities (concurrent with a primary condition) such as asthma or COPD etc.

In the USA a study was carried out *'Prevalence and incidence of noncystic fibrosis bronchiectasis among US adults in 2013'* by *Weycker D. et al and published in Chron Respir Dis 2017 Nov: 14 (4) 377 – 387, Epub 2017, May 30* to try to get a clearer picture of bronchiectasis prevalence, incidence and diagnosis in US clinical practice.

This study used data from 33.2 million adults in the 'MarketScan Database' of private medical healthcare insurance claims. The study's findings included;

- ✓ the most common comorbidities of bronchiectasis, by rank were COPD, acute bronchitis, post-inflammatory fibrosis and genetic disorders
- ✓ prevalence increased with age
- ✓ incidence was higher in women than men and again, increased with age
- ✓ the prevalence of bronchiectasis in the US is higher in adults of all ages than previously thought. The number is between 340,000 and 522,00 with 70,000 adults diagnosed each year. The diagnosis has been growing steadily since 2001 at 8% per annum.

In Germany a study *'Bronchiectasis in Germany: a population- based estimation of disease prevalence'* was prepared by *Ringshausen F.C. et al* and published in the ERS *European Respiratory Journal 2015 46: 1805 -1807.* The aim of this study was to estimate the overall bronchiectasis prevalence in Germany over one year based on a representative sample of statutory health insurance data. People with concomitant COPD were excluded from the analysis upon which the study was based.

It was acknowledged that there was a prior lack of research and that European data was scarce about the condition. Accurate data were important for authorities so that they could allocate appropriate health care resources, especially as bronchiectasis is associated with high healthcare usage as well as having a significant morbidity (extent that two pathological condition exist together) and mortality.

The study's findings included;

- bronchiectasis overall was more common among females than males
- highest prevalence was amongst men aged 75-84 years
- bronchiectasis was estimated at 67 cases per 100,000 population, which extrapolated for a 2013 population of 80.8 million to 54,136 people
- bronchiectasis is not a rare disease in Germany and the prevalence is well above the cut-off figure of 5 per 10,000 for an 'orphan disease' in Europe
- the majority of patients were managed in outpatient care
- 58% of patients presented with chronic airway obstruction; with COPD being the main concomitant diagnosis
- It is likely that, for technical reasons, the study still underestimates the true prevalence of bronchiectasis
- International collaborations will provide additional epidemiology (the study of disease as it affects groups of people, as opposed to individuals) about, in particular, its association with COPD.

In South Korea a study *'Population-based prevalence of bronchiectasis and associated* *comorbidities in South Korea'* was produced by *Choi H. et al* and published in the *ERS European Respiratory Journal, 29 August 2019, 54(2).*

As well as summarising how bronchiectasis occurs and its symptoms, the study's extract states that while bronchiectasis has been regarded as an 'orphan' disease, recent studies have shown that its prevalence (number of cases at a given time) is increasing and that it causes a significant burden on public health including increased healthcare costs, hospital admissions and mortality.

In Catalonia (Spain) a study *'Prevalence and incidence of bronchiectasis in Catalonia in 2012'* was produced by *Fernandez M. B. et al* and published in the ERS *European Respiratory Journal 2016 48: PA667.*

The study's abstract stated that the true incidence (rate of occurrence) and prevalence of non-cystic fibrosis (CF) bronchiectasis were not well known. Accordingly, the study's aims were to determine the prevalence and incidence of bronchiectasis not due to CF in primary care in 2012 in Catalonia, which is a region in Spain, and to describe the clinical characteristics, treatment and health burden of the patients.

Data was obtained from SIDIAP a Catalonian database. Prevalence was estimated from all patients with a codified bronchiectasis diagnosis at 31 December 2012 which totalled 20,895.

Bronchiectasis results included;

- ✓ the overall prevalence and incidence rates for women was higher than for men
- ✓ both prevalence and incidence increased with age in both genders
- ✓ the highest prevalence and incidence were estimated for men aged 65 – 99
- ✓ the mean age was 68.3 years with an equal distribution between genders
- ✓ In the previous year, 55.9% of patients had at least one exacerbation (worsening of bronchiectasis symptoms by infection) and 12.6% were hospitalised.

The study concluded that the prevalence of bronchiectasis in Catalonia increases with age, especially in men aged 65 and over. There is a high use of health resources in bronchiectasis patients.

In Australia and New Zealand possibly the most significant development for bronchiectasis research was the establishment of a critical data platform in Australia in 2015 by the Lung Foundation Australia and the Australasian Bronchiectasis Consortium of the Australian Bronchiectasis Registry (ABR). The ABR (www.bronchiectasis.com.au/registry) was expanded to New Zealand to assist the newly established New Zealand Bronchiectasis Registry.

The Australian Bronchiectasis Consortium has collaborated with both the American Bronchiectasis Registry and the European Bronchiectasis Registry in knowledge, expertise and the optimisation of research outcomes.

The Bronchiectasis Toolbox (www.bronchiectasis.com.au) which is an educational website, contains much useful information about bronchiectasis. It was developed by *Caroline Nicolson* and her article *'The Bronchiectasis Toolbox – A Comprehensive Website for the Management of People with Bronchiectasis'*, pub *Med Sci (Basel) 2017 June; 5 (2): 13 was critically reviewed by A. Holland and A.L. Lee.*

Two valuable Australian reports by *Visser et al* were *'The Management of Bronchiectasis in Adults', Med Journ Aust, Vol 209, issue 4: pages 177-183* and *'Australian Adults with Bronchiectasis: The first report from the Australian Bronchiectasis Registry', Respir Med 155; 2019 Aug: 97-103.*

Recent research into antibiotics treatments for bronchiectasis

Antibiotics for adults

Inhaled antibiotics

A recent review report, based on 135 articles, from South Korea *'Efficacy of inhaled ciprofloxacin agents for the treatment of bronchiectasis; a systematic review and meta-analysis of randomized controlled trials'* by *Jeong U K Lim et al* was published in the *Therapeutic Advances in Respiratory Disease* journal

(20.9 2019). The report's findings found that treatment with inhaled ciprofloxacin medications holds the potential to prevent the acute worsening of respiratory problems in patients with bronchiectasis.

Lung infections have been regarded as the main cause for the worsening of bronchiectasis symptoms/exacerbations. Ciprofloxacin has been effective in treating the pathogen *Pseudomonas aeruginosa* which is one of the more common contributory causes of these exacerbations. However, despite the beneficial effect of this broad - spectrum antibiotic, which contrasts to other types of antibiotic, clinical data suggests that some patients may develop resistance to it, so further long-term studies are required to come to a conclusive therapeutic assessment of ciprofloxacin.

Although inhaled antibiotics have proved effective in cystic fibrosis, most seemed to have failed to benefit bronchiectasis patients. In this Korean study, the team reviewed randomised clinical trials data that evaluated the results of tests on ciprofloxacin and alpulmiq another inhalation antibiotic for non-CF bronchiectasis. Clinical information from 1,685 bronchiectasis trials patients with a follow up of one year was studied and the results showed that inhaled ciprofloxacin significantly prevented exacerbations, the time for a first exacerbation, and severity risk.

While inhaled ciprofloxacin could eradicate harmful pathogens such as *P. aeruginosa* (which can cause severe acute and chronic infections in all parts of the body) from the lungs, results varied between different trials. The team also found that the treatment was linked to a higher risk for emergence of resistance.

It was this seeming contraindication which led to the overall conclusion that while 'inhaled ciprofloxacin showed clinical benefit in terms of pulmonary exacerbations in bronchiectasis patients' given the significance increase of resistance 'clinical trials with a longer study period are required for a conclusive assessment'.

Long term macrolide antibiotics use

A study *'Long- term macrolide antibiotics for the treatment of bronchiectasis in adults: an individual participant data meta-analysis'* by Chalmers J D et al was published online on 9 August 2019 in the journal *'The Lancet Respiratory Medicine'.*

Bronchiectasis treatment guidelines indicate that patients who have three or more exacerbations each year but don't have infection caused by the bacteria *P. aeruginosa* should undergo long term macrolide antibiotic treatment. This type of antibiotic inhibits the growth of bacteria and is used to often treat common bacterial infections.

Although several trials indicated that this treatment prevented bronchiectasis exacerbations this was a small sample which couldn't provide strong conclusions about the effect of such antibiotic treatment in subpopulations of bronchiectasis patients.

An international team of researchers conducted a systematic review and analysis of the benefits of macrolide treatments in the subgroups including those for which macrolide therapy is not currently recommended. It looked at the frequency of exacerbations that required antibiotic treatment; the time to first exacerbation and the changes in quality of life.

The researchers identified controlled clinical trials testing macrolide treatments of adults with bronchiectasis. These patients were divided into subgroups including age, gender, smoking, use of inhaled corticosteroids, BMI, baseline FEV1 and status of *P. aeruginosa.*

They identified 234 studies and patient data from 341 participants in three controlled trials in Australia, New Zealand and the Netherlands. The results indicated that a 6-12 months treatment with macrolides;

- ✓ reduced the frequency of exacerbations by almost 50%
- ✓ increased the time to first exacerbation
- ✓ was associated with an improvement in the quality of life
- ✓ reduced the frequency of exacerbations across all the subgroups
- ✓ there was a high level of treatment benefit with *P. aeruginosa* infections

✓ there was no significant improvement in lung function (as assessed through FEV1).

From these findings the researchers concluded that;

✓ macrolides had a significant impact on patients, in whom macrolides are not considered as a first-line treatment, including those with *P. aeruginosa* and also for those with fewer than three exacerbations annually
✓ macrolides might be considered for patients for whom macrolides are not indicated according to current treatment guidelines; particularly if alternative treatments to reduce exacerbations have been unsuccessful
✓ the longer-term efficacy and safety of macrolides in the bronchiectasis population is unknown, as no studies were discovered with a treatment duration of more than one year
✓ patients and their clinicians should discuss the benefits and risks of macrolides
✓ as macrolides can have adverse effects, such as the potential to induce resistance to antibiotics, they should be used carefully.

Antibiotics for children

A review study '*Which antibiotics should be used to treat children with an acute exacerbation of bronchiectasis and as long-term prevention*' by Gregson E. C was published in the journal '*Archives of Disease in Childhood*' (online 20/7/2019 and in

Volume 104 -10 October 2019 issue) highlighted the lack of data on the use of different antibiotics to treat and/or prevent acute bronchiectasis exacerbations in children and also the need for more research.

While antibiotics are often prescribed for acute bronchiectasis exacerbations it is often not known if one is more effective than another. Researchers found that there were few scientific studies available to answer this important question. Two studies were found that assessed the use of antibiotics to control bronchiectasis exacerbations;

- the first, looked at treatment with amoxicillin-clavulanate & placebo or azithromycin & placebo. While exacerbations were resolved by a similar amount, they were significantly shorter in the amoxicillin group and there was no significant difference in terms of efficacy
- the second, looked at patients positive for bronchiectasis with the bacteria *P aeruginosa*. They randomly received inhaled amikacin and vein intravenous antibiotics; or only intravenous antibiotics. The addition of amikacin more than doubled the rate of bacterial eradication. However, as this type of infection is relatively rare (16%) in bronchiectasis it is questionable to generalise these findings to the bronchiectasis population as a whole.

An additional study was found which assessed the long-term use of antibiotics to reduce children's bronchiectasis exacerbations. 89 Australasian children with either bronchiectasis or chronic suppurative lung disease were treated with azithromycin or a placebo for 1 to 2 years.

While there was a significantly lower frequency of exacerbations in the group treated with azithromycin there was also a higher frequency of bacteria resistance to this antibiotic. These conclusions suggest that long – term use of antibiotics should be followed with caution so as not to generate bacteria resistant to this form of treatment.

Although there are only a few studies in adults, their results can't be extrapolated to children. Additionally, these adults' studies didn't suggest that any one antibiotic might be better than another in treating exacerbations.

Finally, Gregson's review study found that azithromycin while being effective in controlling and /or preventing exacerbations was neither better or worse than others. There is a need for more studies about antibiotic use for children with bronchiectasis.

Immune deficiency research

In a paper by Chalmers J., et al, Dundee University presented at the European Respiratory Society (ERS) 2019 International Congress, Madrid it was found that the protein PZP was present in sputum samples of patients with bronchiectasis or COPD and with lung infections, but not in healthy people. Higher PZP levels also correlated with greater disease severity, more frequent infections, reduced lung function and quality of life. Antibiotic treatment reduced PZP production in the airways of bronchiectasis patients and chest infections. The researchers found that the bacteria causing the lung infections are 'hijacking' the body's defence mechanisms and shielding themselves from the immune system. If the body's natural immune system defence mechanisms can be kickstarted then the cycle of chest infections can be broken.

Lung transplantation for bronchiectasis sufferers

A report *'Outcomes of lung transplantation in adults with bronchiectasis'* by *Birch J, et al.* was published in the journal *BMC pulmonary medicine, 22 May 2018*

An observational study *'The Outcomes of Lung Transplantation in Patients with Bronchiectasis and Antibody Deficiency'* by Nathan J.A, et al. was published in *The Journal of Heart and Lung Transplantation, October 2005, vol 24, issue 10 pages 1517 -1521*

A national cohort study *'Disease- Specific Survival Benefit of Lung Transplantation in Adults'* by Titman A, et al. was published in *the American Journal of Transplantation, Vol 9, issue 7 29 June 2009*

A patient case series study *'Lung transplantation for non – cystic fibrosis bronchiectasis'* by *Rademacher J, et al.* was published in *Respiratory Med. 2016; 115:60 -5.*

Alternative/complementary therapies and nutritional supplements

Whilst complementary/ alternative therapies are often ignored by much of the medical profession, the *British Thoracic Society* in its *2019 Guideline for Bronchiectasis in Adults* contained many recommendations which included;
- ❖ 'that further interventional/ randomised controlled trials are needed to establish the role of any alternative therapies in the management of bronchiectasis' (page 6)
- ❖ 'studies assessing the benefits of nutritional supplementation in patients with bronchiectasis should be undertaken' (page 6).

Currently, many mainstream medical practitioners and researchers are trying to stimulate debate about bronchiectasis especially its causes, symptoms and treatment and which for good reason has been called an 'emerging global epidemic'. An excellent example of this can be found on the ten minute audio by Prof Anne Chang *'Improving the lives of patients with bronchiectasis'* which is linked to the end of the references to the summary of the article *'Bronchiectasis in children: diagnosis and treatment'* by A Chang, A Bush and K Grimwood published in the Lancet Series, Bronchiectasis, vol 392, issue 10150, P866-879, 8.9.2018.

One of the things that has struck me while writing this book are the number of written comments made by leading members of the respiratory sector of the medical and therapy professions about the dearth of solid information which exists about Bronchiectasis and the treatments used to treat it. Examples of this include;

the recent statement given by the British Thoracic Society (BTS) about the commissioning of a new BTS Clinical Statement to be produced in 2020 which will provide guidance on the Assessment and Management of Respiratory Problems in Athletes included;

❖ 'This document will provide much needed guidance for respiratory health care professionals who care for both adults and children with respiratory conditions who wish to pursue sporting activities'.

the *BTS Guideline for Bronchiectasis in Adults published in Thorax journal January 2019 vol 74 Supplement 1* included the following statements;

❖ the need to explore the role of bronchiectasis education, self -management plans and who delivers pulmonary rehabilitation (PR) needs to be explored as does the role of PR after exacerbations requiring hospital admissions' research needs (contained on page 6)

❖ regarding standard laboratory tests; (pages 14-15) it was stated that 'the evidence for the role of aetiological investigations is derived from studies of low to moderate quality' details of other limitations about laboratory tests followed

❖ the BTS Guideline (page 23) recommended that 'Randomised controlled trials using clinically important outcome measures are required to assess the effectiveness of airway clearance techniques in varying severities of bronchiectasis' and 'Randomised controlled trials are required to

evaluate the effects of airway clearance techniques in patients who are undergoing an exacerbation"
- ❖ the BTS Guideline (page 24) states that relating to frequency of airway clearance technique sessions 'there is no evidence to support a particular frequency with recommendations of once or twice daily treatment commonly given'
- ❖ the BTS Guideline (page 27) recommends that 'Randomised, controlled trials are needed to assess the long-term impact of anti-inflammatory therapies
- ❖ the BTS Guideline (page 38) stated that 'there is insufficient evidence to evaluate the efficacy of antibiotics in exacerbations in adults with bronchiectasis'
- ❖ the BTS Guideline (page 44) stated 'There are no studies in bronchiectasis comparing different monitoring schedules, or relating particular monitoring strategies to clinical outcomes'.

In the *BMC Pulmonary Medicine journal of 22.5.2018* the following statements were included;
- ❖ 'Bronchiectasis has an increasing profile within respiratory medicine. This chronic and irreversible airways disease is common but suffers from a lack of evidence -based therapy for patients and a lack of understanding of its inherent heterogeneity. There is an urgent need for sustained investment into focused, dedicated and collaborative research platforms into bronchiectasis, an emerging 'global epidemic"
- ❖ 'significant knowledge gaps persist in key areas of disease including aetiology, pathogenesis and microbial infection'.

In the *'European Respiratory Society guidelines for the management of adult bronchiectasis'* published in the ERS Journal 2017 50: 1700629 the following statements were included;

❖ 'to date, there are no international guidelines for the management of adult bronchiectasis published and no national guidelines published in the past 5 years'

❖ 'we suggest acute exacerbations of bronchiectasis should be treated with 14 days of antibiotics (*conditional recommendation, very low quality of evidence*).

Printed in Great Britain
by Amazon